Atlas of Gynecologic
PATHOLOGY

Atlas of Gynecologic
PATHOLOGY

Ossama Tawfik MD PhD
Professor of Pathology
Department of Pathology and Laboratory Medicine
The University of Kansas School of Medicine
Kansas City, Kansas

Fang Fan MD PhD
Assistant Professor of Pathology
Department of Pathology and Laboratory Medicine
The University of Kansas School of Medicine
Kansas City, Kansas

Ivan Damjanov MD PhD
Professor of Pathology
Department of Pathology and Laboratory Medicine
The University of Kansas School of Medicine
Kansas City, Kansas

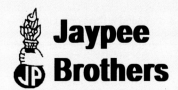
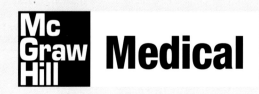

© 2007 Ossama Tawfik, Fang Fan, Ivan Damjanov

First published in India by

Jaypee Brothers Medical Publishers (P) Ltd
EMCA House, 23/23B Ansari Road, Daryaganj, New Delhi 110 002, India
Phones: +91-11-23272143, +91-11-23272703, +91-11-23282021, +91-11-23245672
Fax: +91-11-23276490, +91-11-23245683   e-mail: jaypee@jaypeebrothers.com
Visit our website: www.jaypeebrothers.com

First published in USA by The McGraw-Hill Companies, 2 Penn Plaza, New York, NY 10121-2298. Exclusively worldwide distributor except South Asia (India, Nepal, Sri Lanka, Bhutan, Pakistan, Bangladesh).

NOTICE

Medicine is an ever-changing science. As new research and clinical experience broaden our knowledge, changes in treatment and drug therapy are required. The authors and the publisher of this work have checked with sources believed to be reliable in their efforts to provide information that is complete and generally in accord with the standards accepted at the time of publication. However, in view of the possibility of human error changes in medical science, neither the editors nor the publisher nor any other party who has been involved in the preparation or publication of this work warrants that the information contained herein is in every respect accurate or complete, and they disclaim all responsibility for any errors or omissions or for the results obtained from use of the information contained in this work. Readers are encouraged to confirm the information contained herein with other sources. For example and in particular, readers are advised to check the product information sheet included in the package of each drug they plan to administer to be certain that the information contained in this work is accurate and that changes have not been made in the recommended dose or in the contraindications for administration. This recommendation is of particular importance in connection with new or infrequently used drugs.

ISBN   0-07-148572-4
ISBN 13 9780071485722

PREFACE

Pathology is the basis of clinical medicine. We think that this is a given, and as one of the founders of modern medicine Sir William Osler said, our clinical skills will be only as good as our understanding of pathology. It is thus imperative that we continue to study the anatomic manifestations of diseases and correlate our observations with other manifestations of the same pathological processes in clinics and the laboratory. Modern clinical medicine cannot exist without the support of pathology and laboratory medicine and that is the main reason that all medical students and residents in almost all clinical specialties are expected to learn the basics of pathology as it pertains to their disciplines.

Keeping in mind the postulates listed above we have prepared a brief Atlas of gynecologic pathology. We have compiled it for practicing gynecologists, but we hope that it will be mostly used by gynecologists in training, i.e. residents or registrars or fellows. Most gynecology training programs include gynecologic pathology as a requirement and many gynecologists in training even rotate through pathology departments. This short book, that could be read cover to cover during such a rotation could serve as a comprehensive introduction to gynecologic pathology and would definitely provide enough factual knowledge to pass the specialty Boards.

Over many years we have been teaching clinicians in training and medical students gynecologic pathology. We are thus fairly confident that we know what is important for them to know, what challenges them the most, and what are the pathologic entities that puzzle them the most in their daily practice as well during the intense study time while preparing for the examinations. We hope that this book will help them better understand gynecologic pathology and allow them to correlate the pathologic findings with the clinical data.

Since we are pathologist, we hope that our own residents will also read this book to understand which aspects of pathology are of special clinical significance. One day they might even use it to teach pathology to the next generation of young gynecologists.

Our book is divided into seven chapters covering the pathology of the six principal parts of the female genital tract and the placenta. We have followed the time-tested format of our lectures and have in our presentation included the following elements:

- Review of basic anatomy and histology
- Brief overview of the essential pathology
- Essential background information for the diseases to be illustrated
- Summary of clinical data
- Classification of diseases, whenever needed
- Summary of gross and microscopic pathology
- Representative color illustrations of macroscopic and microscopic pathology.

Each chapter begins with a brief review or the relevant anatomy and histology. With the help of our expert medical illustrator Erica R. Grindle, who is also a student in the program for Pathology Assistants, we have also prepared some semi-schematic drawings of normal anatomy. The text is presented mostly in form of boxed tables and the narrative was reduced to bare minimum. To facilitate the understanding of illustrations we have marked up or annotated most figures. The figures of macroscopic findings were juxtaposed to those of microscopic findings for easy correlation of gross and histologic appearances of the same diseases. The important aspects of many diseases are marked with asterisks and labeled as "pearls".

We hope that the book will be read worldwide and we await eagerly the feedback from our readers. All comments are welcome but especially constructive criticism or suggestions for improvement. Please do not hesitate to send your correspondence by e-mail (otawfik@kumc.edu).

This book would not have been possible without the help of our Chair, Dr. Patricia Thomas, our colleagues and residents in the Department of Pathology, as well our clinician friends at the University of Kansas Hospital. Mr. Dennis Friesen, our departmental photographer provided invaluable help with the color figures. Mr JP Vij, Chairman and Managing Director, Jaypee Brothers Medical Publishers (P) Ltd., New Delhi, encouraged us to start this project and his expert staff, provided the technical support and completed the project in record time. We thank them all.

Kansas City

Ossama Tawfik
Fang Fan
Ivan Damjanov

CONTENTS

Vulva

NORMAL ANATOMY AND HISTOLOGY

Vulva represents the external part of the female genital organs. It consists of the *mons pubis, the labia majora and labia minora, the clitoris, and the vestibule of the vagina* (Fig. 1.1). Vulva includes the external orifice of the urethra and the accessory mucous glands.

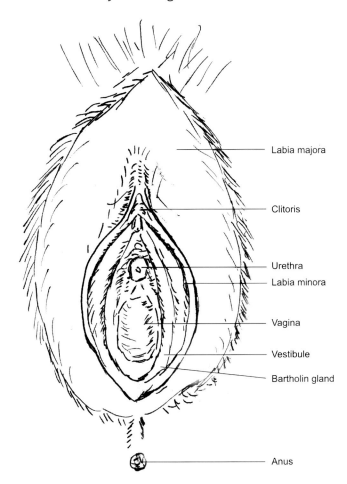

Labia majora

Clitoris

Urethra
Labia minora

Vagina

Vestibule

Bartholin gland

Anus

Figure 1.1. Normal vulva.

The aspects of normal anatomy and histology that are most important for the understanding of vulvar pathology are as follows:

- The vulva is covered with *skin* that is similar to the skin on other parts of the body.
  - Many vulvar diseases are similar to skin diseases affecting other parts of the body.
- Vulvar skin is partially covered with *pubic hair* which covers the mons pubis and lateral sides of the labia majora.
  - Infections of the hair follicles of the pubic area are similar to infections of other hairy parts of the body.
- Histologically, the skin covering the vulva is composed of squamous epithelium. The *squamous epithelium* of the mons pubis, labia majora and minora undergoes surface keratinization (Fig. 1.2).
  - Squamous epithelium is resistant to bacterial infections but can be infected by viruses (e.g. Human popillomavirus—HPV) or fungi (e.g. *Candida albicans*).
  - Most of the tumors of the vulva are squamous cell neoplasms.
- Epithelium covering the vestibule is continuous with the epithelium of vaginal mucosa, which is also a hormone sensitive squamous epithelium. Vulvar mucosa resembles vaginal epithelium and does not show keratinization.
  - Keratinization of vestibular mucosal squamous epithelium is an abnormal finding.
- The vaginal vestibule contains tubular and alveolar glands, the most important of which are the major vestibular glands–*vulvovaginal (Bartholin) and periurethral (Skene) glands*.
  - Bacteria can enter the ducts and infect the glandular epithelium (e.g. Bartholin's gland abscess).
- The vulva is closely related to the terminal parts of the urinary and gastrointestinal tract (anus).
  - Vulvar infections are often related to bacteria from the anus or lower urinary tract.

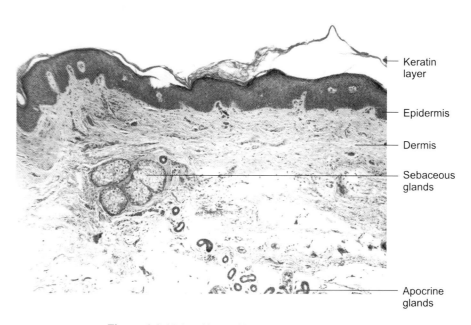

Figure 1.2. Vulva: Normal histology.

OVERVIEW OF PATHOLOGY

The most important diseases of the vulva are classified as follows:

- Inflammatory diseases
- Cysts
- Neoplastic diseases

Inflammatory Diseases

Inflammatory diseases may be infectious, immune-mediated, related to mechanical factors or exogenous irritants, or may have no identifiable causes (Box 1.1).

1. *Infections of vulva:* These can occur in an isolated form or together with involvement of the entire female genital tract or the entire body (Box 1.2).
2. *Genital herpes:* It is the most common sexually transmitted disease of the vulva. Typically, it presents in form of small grouped vesicles. Fluid accumulates inside the tissue clefts formed inside the epithelium (Fig. 1.3). These vesicles tend to recur and usually ulcerate and heal without scarring.
3. *Condyloma acuminatum or genital wart:* It is a exophytic epithelial lesion related to HPV infection. Condylomata lata are usually caused by HPV-6, and less commonly by HPV-11. Like other HPV viruses, these two DNA viruses cause proliferation of squamous epithelium with koilocytic changes (Fig. 1.4). Condylomata acuminata do not progress to neoplasia.
4. *Hidradenitis suppurativa:* It is a bacterial infection of the apocrine glands attached to the hairy part of the vulva (Fig. 1.5).
5. *Non-neoplastic epithelial disorders:* These include several chronic vulvar diseases of noninfectious origin that are classified as follows:
   - *Lichen sclerosus:* This disease of unknown etiology accounts for approximately one-third of all vulvar nonneoplastic chronic diseases (Box 1.3 and Fig. 1.6).
   - *Squamous cell hyperplasia:* It usually presents clinically as a leukoplakia or erythroplakia and could be mistaken for carcinoma (Box 1.4 and Fig. 1.7).
   - *Chronic vulvar dermatitis:* This group of diseases includes many forms of systemic dermatitis such as psoriasis or lichen planus. Histologically, these diseases produce the same change as in the skin of other parts of the body.

Box 1.1. Classification of inflammatory diseases of the vulva

INFECTIOUS DISEASES
- Sexually transmitted diseases
- Urinary tract diseases
- Anal and intestinal diseases
- Skin infections

IMMUNE-MEDIATED DISEASES
- Autoimmune diseases (e.g. pemphigus, bullous pemphigoid)
- Contact allergies (e.g. hypersensitivity to deodorants or hygienic lotions)

MECHANICAL INJURIES AND IRRITATIONS
- Acute injury (e.g. intercourse or delivery-related)
- Chronic irritants (e.g. garment, chemicals)

DISEASES OF UNKNOWN ETIOLOGY

Box 1.2. Infections of the vulva

VIRAL INFECTIONS
- Herpes simplex infection
- Human papilloma virus (HPV) infection

BACTERIAL INFECTIONS
- Gonorrhea
- Syphilis
- Infections with uropathogens/saprophytes

FUNGAL INFECTIONS
- Candidiasis

PARASITES
- Lice infection of pubic hair

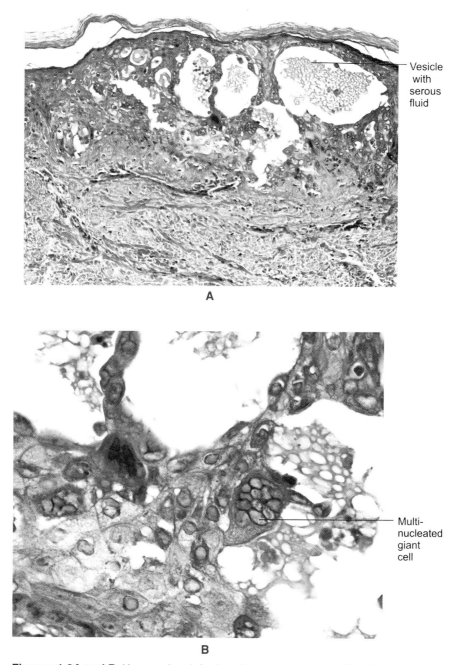

Vesicle
with
serous
fluid

A

Multi-
nucleated
giant
cell

B

Figures 1.3A and B. Herpes virus infection: A. Low-power view of an intraepidermal herpetic vesicle. B. Higher power view of a cluster of multinucleated giant cells with typical intranuclear inclusions.

Fibrous core   Epithelial cells

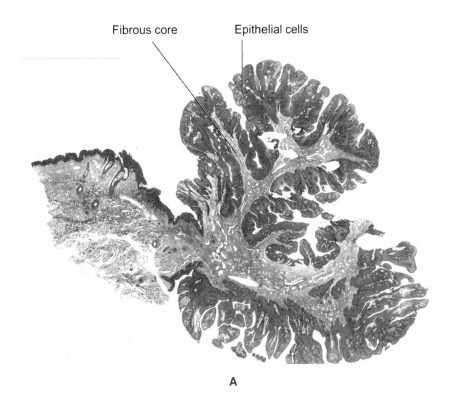

A

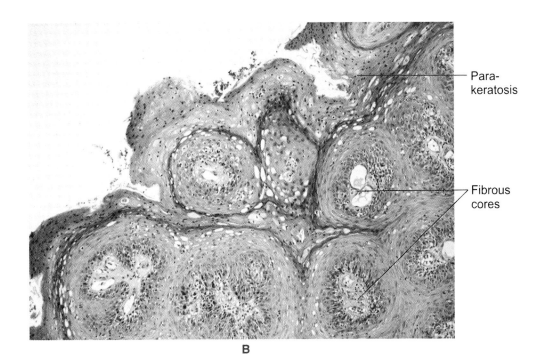

Para-
keratosis

Fibrous
cores

B

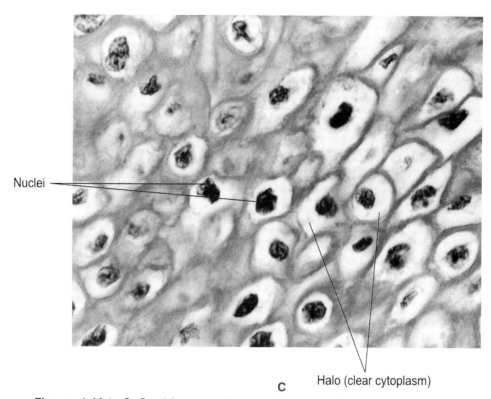

Nuclei

Halo (clear cytoplasm)

C

Figures 1.4A to C. Condyloma acuminatum of vulva: A. The lesion is characterized by papillomatosis, acanthosis and hyperkeratosis. B. Prominent acanthosis and hyperkeratosis. C. Typical koilocytes are noted with raisinoid hyperchromatic nuclei surrounded by a perinuclear cytoplasmic halo.

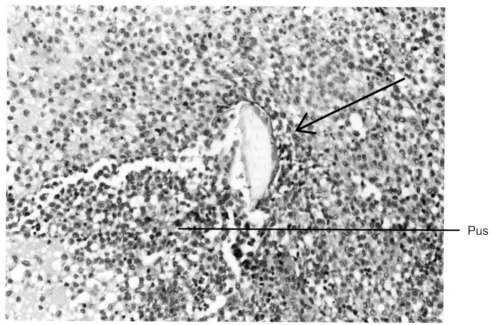

Pus

Figure 1.5. Hidradenitis suppurativa: Extensive marked acute and chronic inflammation in dermis and subcutaneous tissue with abscess formation and a trapped hair shaft (arrow).

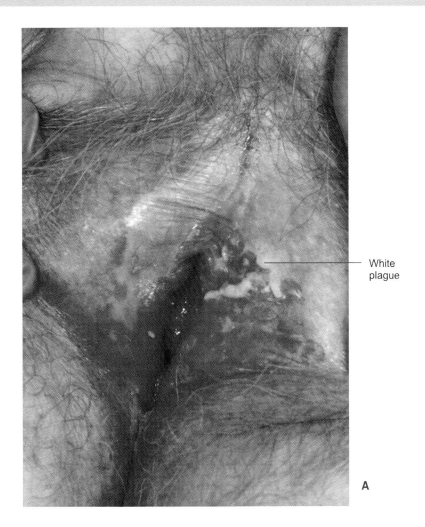

A

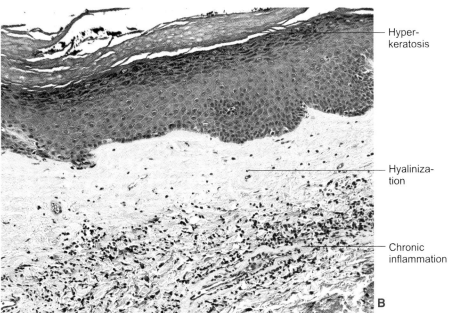

B

Figures 1.6A and B. Lichen sclerosus: A. The vulva is focally covered with pale white plaque-like lesions with focal ecchymosis and ulceration. B. Microscopic features include hyperkeratosis with a loss of rete ridges, subepidermal homogenized zone of edema and hyalinization, and a band of chronic inflammation.

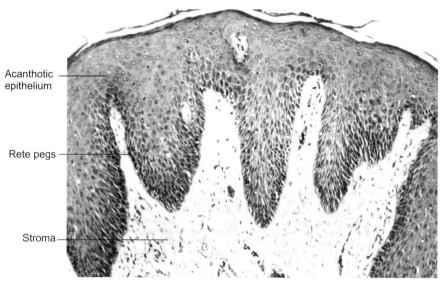

Figure 1.7. Squamous cell hyperplasia (keratosis): The microscopic features include epithelial thickening with acanthosis, hyperkeratosis, and a prominence of the stratum granulosum. Note the absence of nuclear atypia. Mitoses are sparse and limited to the basal layer.

Box 1.3. Lichen sclerosus

CLINICAL FEATURES
- Predominantly in postmenopausal women,* but may occur at any age, even in children
- Intractable itching, soreness, easy bruising
- Initially, red patches that become white plaques
- Skin atrophy ("parchment-like" skin)
- Usually symmetrical, may involve anus ("figure 8"-like)

HISTOPATHOLOGY
- Atrophy of epidermis (loss of rete ridges)
- Hyperkeratosis
- Acellular zone of subepithelial hyalinized collagen
- Chronic inflammation may be seen in deeper dermis.

Pearl: May predispose to cancer—suspicious areas must be biopsied

Box 1.4. Squamous cell hyperplasia

CLINICAL FEATURES
- Itching, dyspareunia
- Leukoplakia (white patch)
- Erythroplakia (red patch)

HISTOPATHOLOGY
- Thickened epithelium, hyperkeratosis, prominent stratum granulosum
- No significant atypia*
- Mild dermal chronic inflammation

Pearl: Epithelium does not show any atypia—a fact important for distinguishing squamous cell hyperplasia from squamous cell dysplasia and carcinoma *in situ*.

CYSTS

Cysts develop from embryonic remnants, invagination of the epidermis, or due to an obstruction of the vulvar gland ducts.

1. *Epidermoid cysts:* These are the most common vulvar cysts. These cysts are similar to those occur in the other parts of the body. They are lined by squamous epithelium and filled with keratinous debris.

2. *Bartholin gland cyst:* It results from obstruction of the major duct (Box 1.5 and Fig. 1.8). Despite the obstruction, the glands continue secreting mucus that accumulates inside the cyst. It occurs chiefly during the reproductive ages.

Neoplastic Diseases

1. *Vulvar intraepithelial neoplasia (VIN):* It represents a spectrum of squamous intraepithelial lesions of the vulvar skin characterized by disordered squamous maturation, nuclear abnormalities, and mitotic figures (Box 1.6). VIN is almost invariably associated with human papillomavirus infection, most commonly HPV type 16.

   The degree of atypia and dysplasia of VIN is pathologically graded as mild, moderate or severe. In VIN 1, atypia is confined to the lower third of the epithelium (Fig. 1.9). In VIN 2, atypia involves the basal and middle thirds of the epithelium (Fig. 1.10).

   In VIN 3, the atypia involves the entire thickness of the epithelium (Fig. 1.11). The lesions may be classified as *warty*, showing surface keratinization and papillomatosis, or *basaloid*, when flat and showing intraepithelial changes similar to those in the cervix.

2. *Invasive squamous cell carcinoma:* It is the most common malignant tumor of the vulva (Box 1.7) and occurs more frequently in older women. Typically, it evolves in the background of VIN. The tumor is composed of invasive squamous cells of varying degrees of differentiation (Figs 1.12 to 1.19 and Box 1.8).

   The prognosis depends on the stage of the tumor and the presence or absence of metastases. Other parameters such as histologic grade, type, and DNA ploidy are also included in the pathology report as they carry certain prognostic significance.

3. *Extramammary Paget's disease:* It is an intraepithelial carcinoma characterized by distinctive large malignant cells growing along the epidermal basal layer (Fig. 1.20). It presents clinically as red and eczematoid lesions resemble dermatosis. In contrast to mammary Paget's disease (typically associated with underlying ductal carcinoma), ductal or glandular carcinoma can rarely be demonstrated underneath the epithelium involved by Paget's disease of the female genital tract. It may histologically resemble malignant melanoma, which must be excluded before the diagnosis of extramammary Paget's disease is made.

Box 1.5. Bartholin's gland cyst

PATHOGENESIS
- Duct obstruction by secretions
- Infection with scarring/obstruction

CLINICAL FEATURES
- Painful swelling
- Tenderness
- Occurs mostly during reproductive age

HISTOPATHOLOGY
- Cyst lining—transitional epithelium
- Cyst wall—fibrous tissue, atrophic acini and some chronic inflammatory cells

THERAPY
- Incision, drainage, antibiotics.

Box 1.6. Vulvar intraepithelial neoplasia (VIN)

CLINICAL FEATURES
- Maybe asymptomatic
- Vulvar pruritus or irritation
- Macular or papular lesion, maybe pigmented

HISTOPATHOLOGY
- Warty pattern of VIN*
- Basaloid pattern of VIN*

*Note: Lesions are graded histologically as VIN 1, VIN 2 or VIN 3

Box 1.7. Epidemiology of squamous cell carcinoma of the vulva

- Old age disease (mean age at diagnosis—65 years)
- Less common than other gynecologic cancer
- Accounts for only 5% of gynecologic cancers
- Incidence has not increased over the last 20 years
- Some related to HPV, but most are not

Mucous glands

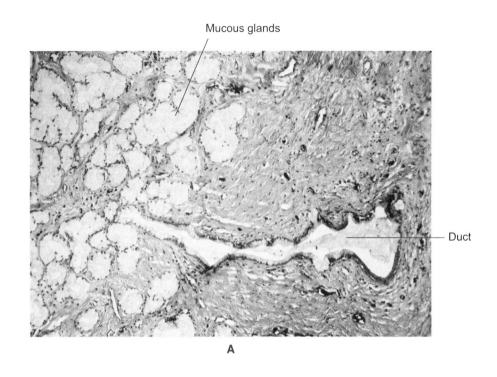

Duct

A

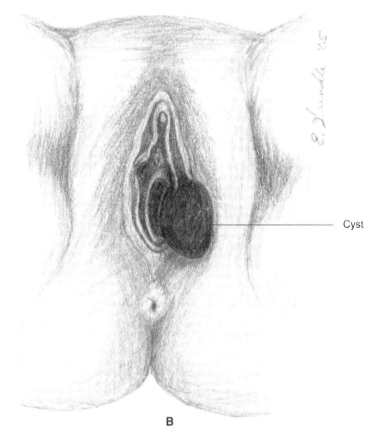

Cyst

B

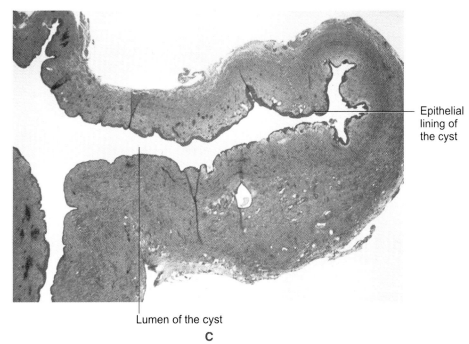

Epithelial
lining of
the cyst

Lumen of the cyst

C

Figures 1.8A to C. Bartholin's gland and Bartholin's gland cyst: A. The normal gland is composed of mucous glands and excretory ducts. B. Bartholin's gland cyst. It is located in labia minora and forms a protruding mass. Obstruction of the duct is accompanied by inflammation, imparting the inflamed cyst a red color. C. Microscopically, the cyst is lined by transitional or squamous epithelium.

Box 1.8. Clinical pathologic features of squamous carcinoma of the vulva

CLINICAL FEATURES
- Pruritus, bleeding, infection
- Plaque, ulcer, mass

MACROSCOPIC PATHOLOGY
- Exophytic (70%)
- Ulcerative
- Endophytic

HISTOPATHOLOGIC TYPES
- Keratinizing invasive squamous cell carcinoma (KISCC)*
- Warty invasive squamous cell carcinoma (WISCC)
- Basaloid invasive squamous cell carcinoma (BISCC)

METASTASES
- Inguinal lymph nodes, followed by iliac lymph nodes.

Pearls: KISCC is the most common and accounts for 65% of all tumors.

WISCC and BISCC in younger women may be related to HPV infection, but KISCC (usually in older women) is not.

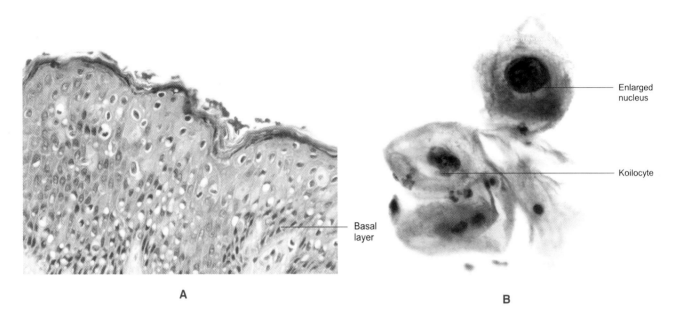

A

B

Figures 1.9A and B. Vulvar intraepithelial neoplasia 1 (VIN 1): A. Squamous dysplasia is minimal and limited to the basal layers of epithelium. Koilocytes are signs of HPV infection. B. Cytologic smear of low grade intraepithelial neoplasia contains cells that have enlarged, hyperchromatic nuclei and show koilocytic features.

4. *Melanocytic tumors:* These include benign melanocytic nevi and malignant melanomas.
   - *Melanocytic nevus:* Congenital and acquired nevi (moles) occur in the vulva, usually in the labia majora. These nevi have the same features as nevi in other locations (Fig. 1.21).
   - *Malignant melanoma:* This rare tumor accounts for 5 to 10% of vulvar malignancies and is the second most common malignant tumor at this site. Pathologically, it has the same features as skin melanomas in other sites (Box 1.9 and Figs 1.21 to 1.23).

5. *Mesenchymal tumors and tumor-like lesions:* They are rare. The most important lesions are as follows:
   - *Fibroepithelial polyp:* This superficially located polypoid vulvar lesion is composed of loose myxoid stroma covered by normal squamous epithelium (Fig. 1.24).
   - *Aggressive angiomyxoma:* This tumor often presents as a bulky vulvar mass no sharp margins. The mean age at diagnosis is 30 years, but the tumor may also occur in older or younger women, and even in children. Clinically, it mimics a Bartholin's gland cyst or hernia. The tumor is composed of spindle or stellate shaped cells arranged in myxoid stroma around thin-walled and thick-walled blood vessels (Fig. 1.25). These cells have immunohistochemical features characteristic of smooth muscle cells.

Box 1.9. Malignant melanoma of the vulva

CLINICAL FEATURES
- Postmenopausal women (50-70 years)
- Pruritus, bleeding, dysuria, dyspareunia

MACROSCOPIC PATHOLOGY
- Pigmented or nonpigmented mass
- Often ulcerated, friable, necrotic
- Cutaneous satellite nodules may be present

HISTOPATHOLOGY
- Large pleomorphic cells with irregular nuclei and prominent nucleoli
- Junctional activity and spread of melanocytes; mitoses evident
- Upward migration of melanocytes in epidermis and invasion of dermis
- Variable melanin pigmentation
- Immunohistochemical stains useful: S-100 (+), Melan A (+), HMB45 (+).

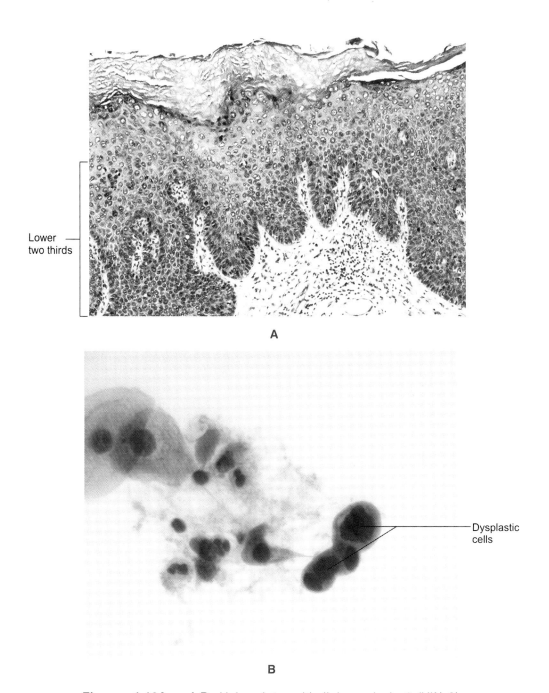

Lower
two thirds

A

Dysplastic
cells

B

Figures 1.10A and B. Vulvar intraepithelial neoplasia 2 (VIN 2):
A. Squamous dysplasia involves the lower two thirds of the epithelial layer,
which also shows marked koilocytic changes and scattered mitoses.
B. Pap smear shows dysplastic squamous cells with a high nuclear-
cytoplasmic ratio and hyperchromatic nuclei.

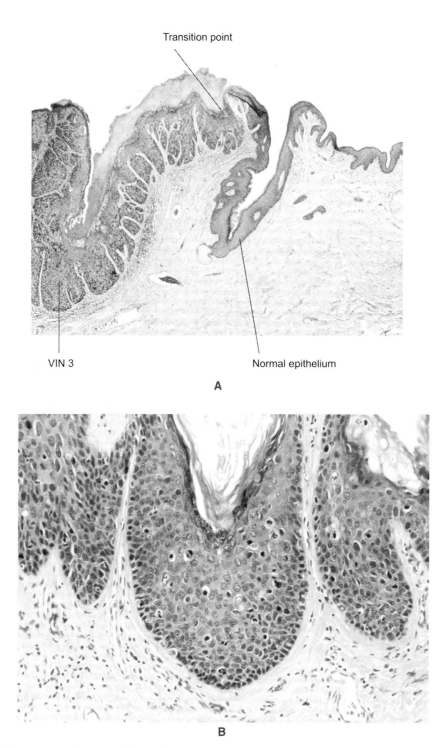

Transition point

VIN 3   Normal epithelium

A

B

Figures 1.11A and B. Vulvar intraepithelial neoplasia 3 (VIN 3): A. Low-power view showing the transition between normal and dysplastic epithelium. Notice the full thickness dysplasia of the epithelium and the absence of stromal invasion. B. High-power view showing loss of normal maturation, nuclear pleomorphism, hyperchromasia, and increased mitotic activity throughout the entire thickness of epithelium.

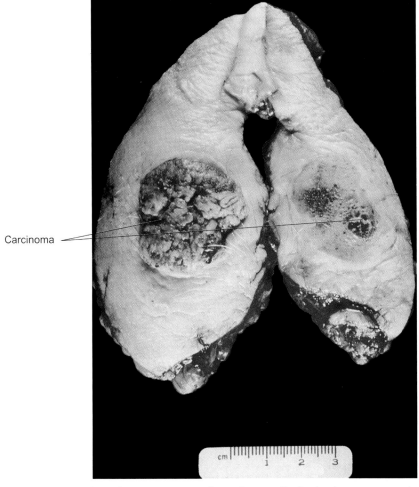

Carcinoma

Figure 1.12. Invasive squamous cell carcinoma. Radical vulvectomy specimen showing bilateral fungating ulcerative lesions on both sides of the vulva.

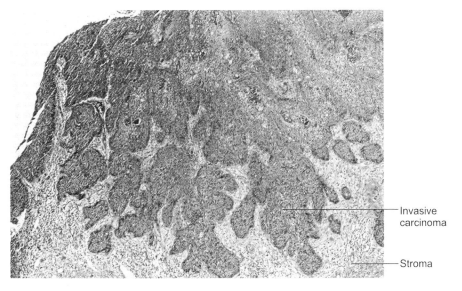

Invasive carcinoma

Stroma

Figure 1.13. Invasive squamous cell carcinoma of vulva: The tumor shows marked stromal invasion. The tumor thickness is measured from the surface or the granular layer of epithelium to the deepest point of invasion. The depth of invasion is measured from the epithelial stromal junction of the adjacent most superficial dermal papillae to the deepest point of invasion.

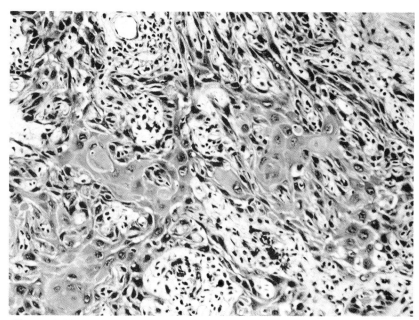

Figure 1.14. Well-differentiated, invasive squamous cell carcinoma of vulva. The tumor is keratinized and shows moderate nuclear atypia.

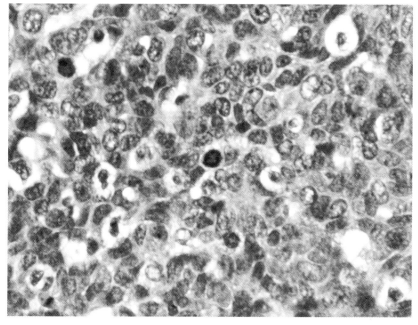

Figure 1.15. Poorly-differentiated, invasive non-keratinizing squamous cell carcinoma of vulva. Sheets of anaplastic tumor cells show no keratinization.

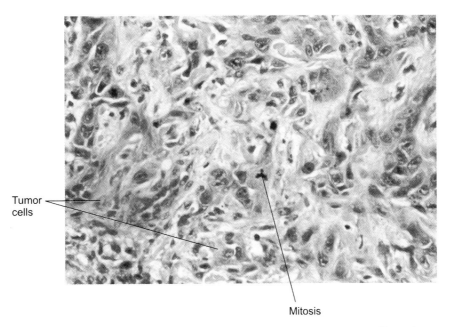

Tumor cells

Mitosis

Figure 1.16. Poorly-differentiated, invasive keratinizing squamous cell carcinoma of vulva. Sheets of anaplastic tumor cells evoke a desmoplastic stromal response. Individual cell keratinization is present.

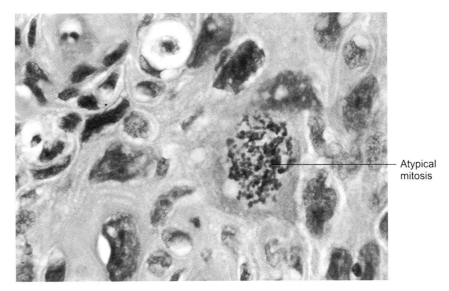

Atypical mitosis

Figure 1.17. Poorly-differentiated, invasive non-keratinizing squamous cell carcinoma of vulva. High-power view shows marked anaplasia and frequent atypical mitosis.

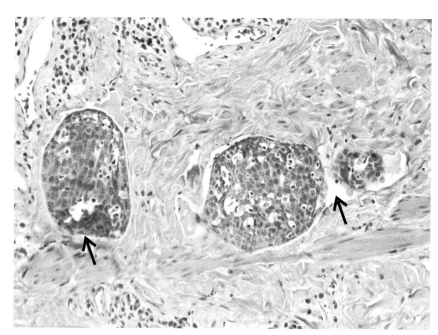

Figure 1.18. Poorly-differentiated, invasive non-keratinizing squamous cell carcinoma of vulva. Lymphatic spaces contain tumor cells (arrow).

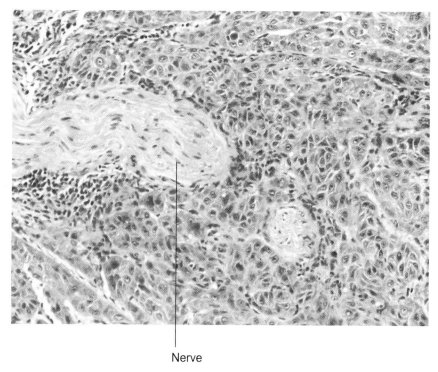

Nerve

Figure 1.19. Moderately-differentiated, invasive keratinizing squamous cell carcinoma of vulva. There is perineural invasion by tumor cells.

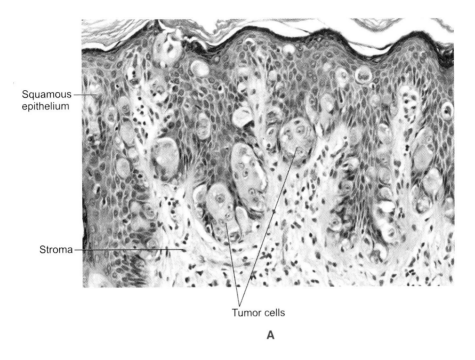

Squamous epithelium

Stroma

Tumor cells

A

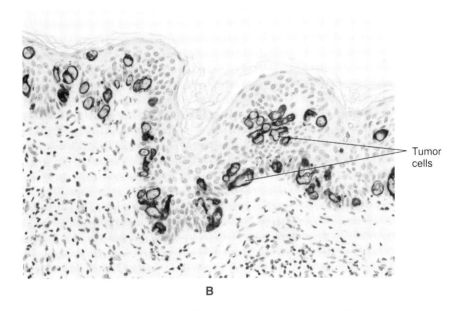

Tumor cells

B

Figures 1.20A and B. Extramammary Paget's disease of vulva: A. The epidermis contains groups of cells and single large pale tumor cells that differ from the surrounding squamous cells. B. Immunohistochemical stain for epithelial membrane antigen (EMA) highlights the Paget's cells in the epidermis.

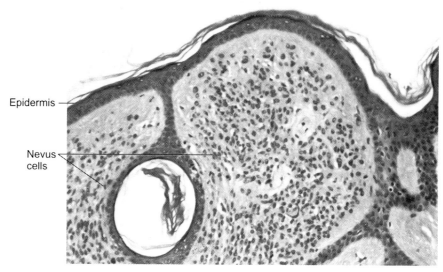

Epidermis —

Nevus cells —

Figure 1.21. Intradermal nevus: Benign melanocytic nevus cells are noted in the dermis.

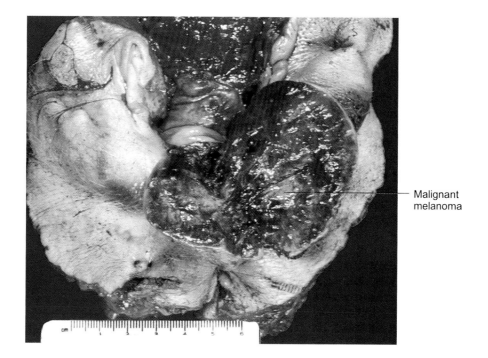

— Malignant melanoma

Figure 1.22. Radical vulvectomy specimen with malignant melanoma: The tumor shows areas of brown pigmentation, hemorrhage, and necrosis. The green ink was added during dissection to indicate the visible margins of this tumor.

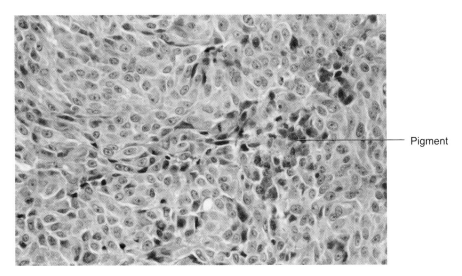

Figure 1.23. Malignant melanoma of vulva: Sheets of large malignant cells with atypical nuclei and prominent nucleoli. Occasional melanin pigmentation is seen.

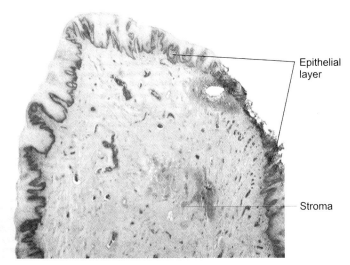

Figure 1.24. Fibroepithelial polyp: The lesion is composed of benign squamous epithelium and benign fibrovascular stroma. The epidermis shows with no cellular atypia or koilocytic changes.

- *Angiomyofibroblastoma:* This rare benign vulvar tumor usually presents as a well-demarcated small nodule measuring less than 5 cm in diameter. It is composed of thin-walled blood vessels surrounded by rings of spindle-shaped cells bordered by less cellular acellular spaces (Fig. 1.26). The spindle cells are epithelioid myofibroblasts, which have eosinophilic cytoplasm and stain immunohistochemically with antibodies to smooth muscle markers (e.g. desmin or smooth muscle cell actin).

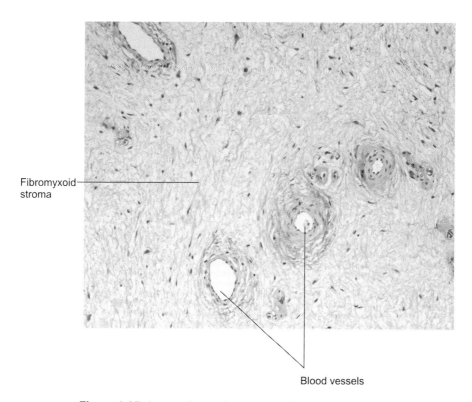

Fibromyxoid stroma

Blood vessels

Figure 1.25. Aggressive angiomyxoma of vulva: Hypocellular fibromyxoid stroma contains prominent medium-sized blood vessels.

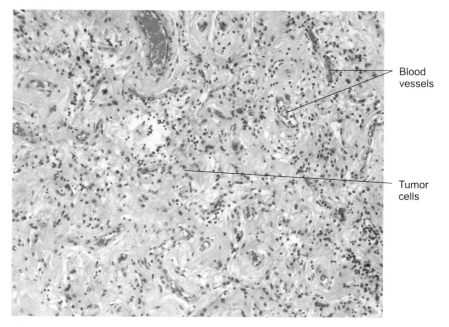

Blood vessels

Tumor cells

Figure 1.26. Angiomyofibroblastoma of vulva: The tumor is moderately cellular and consists of spindle-shaped myofibroblasts surrounded by fibrotic extracellular matrix. There are scattered small blood vessels.

- *Angiosarcoma:* This form of sarcoma rarely occurs in the vulva. It is usually hemorrhagic and necrotic and bleeds easily. It is composed of malignant endothelial cells and is similar to angiosarcomas in other locations (Fig. 1.27).

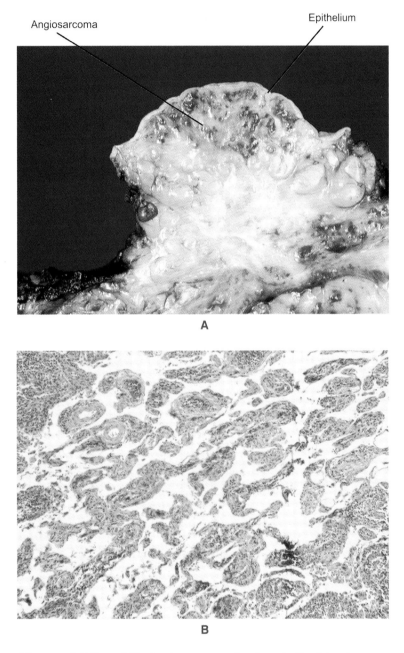

Figures 1.27A and B. Angiosarcoma of vulva: A. Partial vulvectomy specimen with a cross-section showing dermal and subcutaneous tissue involvement by a hemorrhagic ill-defined tumor. B. There are numerous vascular spaces lined by large atypical malignant endothelial cells.

2

Vagina

NORMAL ANATOMY AND HISTOLOGY

Vagina is a tubular structure that extends from the vulvar vestibule to the uterine cervix. It lies anterior to the rectum and posterior to the urinary bladder and urethra (Fig. 2.1). The uterine cervix protrudes into the upper vagina thus forming the vaginal fornix; a recess between the uterine cervix and the lateral wall of the upper vagina.

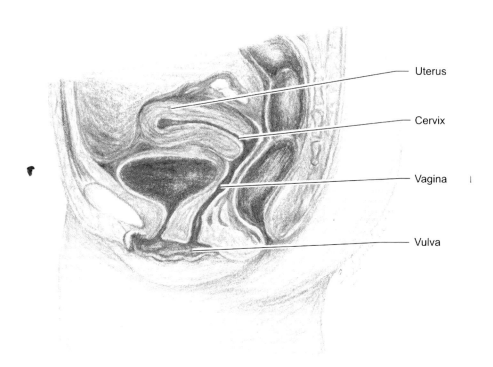

Figure 2.1. Normal vagina: It is located anterior to the rectum and posterior to the urinary bladder and urethra. It extends from the vulva to the cervix of the uterus.

The vagina is covered with nonkeratinizing squamous epithelium, which is continuous with the epithelium of the vulva on one side and the epithelium of the cervix on the other. The most important aspects of vaginal histology that are useful for the understanding of vaginal pathology are as follows:

- The vaginal wall is composed of three layers: *mucosa, muscularis and adventitia.*
    - The vagina does not have a serosa and accordingly tumors that have reached the adventitia easily invade the adjacent organs.
- The vagina is lined by *stratified nonkeratinizing squamous epithelium.* This epithelium is divided into distinct layers, which include basal, parabasal, intermediate and superficial layers (Fig. 2.2A).
    - Irregular maturation of squamous epithelium results in squamous dysplasia.
    - The severity of squamous dysplasia is graded according to extent of involvement of various layers of the epithelium.
- The thickness of the epithelium varies depending on *the age of the woman and her hormonal status.* Before menarche the epithelium is thin with little evidence of maturation. After puberty, the thickness of the epithelium increases as a result of cellular proliferation and maturation. After menopause, the epithelium is reduced to only a few layers of parabasal and basal cells (Fig. 2.2B).
    - The lack of estrogen after menopause accounts for the atrophy of the epithelium, which is more vulnerable to trauma and less resistant to infection.
- Maturation of vaginal squamous epithelium includes accumulation of *glycogen* in the intermediate and superficial layers. Glycogen-rich cells desquamating into the lumen of the vagina are the source of glycogen, which is metabolized into *lactic acid* the by intravaginal bacilli.
    - Lactic acid and the thickness of the epithelium provide a *barrier to infection* in adult women; such infections are more common in premenarchal and postmenopausal vaginas.
- The squamous epithelium of the vaginal mucosa is in continuity with the ectocervical mucosa.
    - Vaginal and cervical squamous cell carcinomas have identical histologic features. Actually, the most common vaginal carcinomas are cervical carcinomas extending into the vagina.

The vagina develops from two primordia: the upper vagina develops from the mullerian ducts and the lower vagina develops from the urogenital sinus. Incomplete caudal development and fusion of the lower part of the mullerian ducts result in congenital *absence of vagina* (Fig. 2.3). The patients with this congenital anomaly have normal external genitalia but the vagina is missing and is replaced by a short blind pouch. *Septate vagina* is another rare congenital anomaly resulting from incomplete fusion of the müllerian ducts. It is characterized by a longitudinal septum dividing the vagina into two compartments (Fig. 2.4). Clinically, this anomaly usually remains asymptomatic.

OVERVIEW OF PATHOLOGY

The most important diseases of the vagina are classified as follows:
- Non-neoplastic lesions
- Neoplasms

Non-neoplastic Lesions

1. *Vaginal adenosis:* It refers to the presence of aberrant glandular elements in the vaginal mucosa. It is typically found in young women who were exposed *in utero* to diethylstilbestrol (DES). Clinically, vaginal adenosis may present with excessive mucus discharge. By colposcopy one may find red granular mucosal spots. Microscopically,

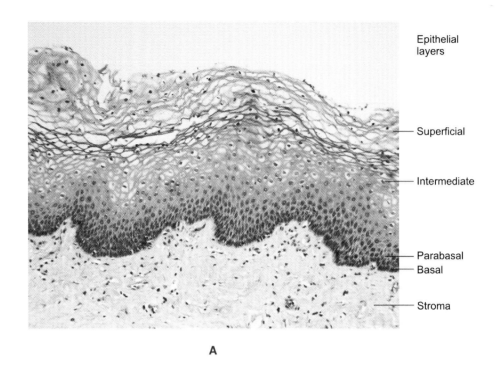

Epithelial
layers

Superficial

Intermediate

Parabasal
Basal

Stroma

A

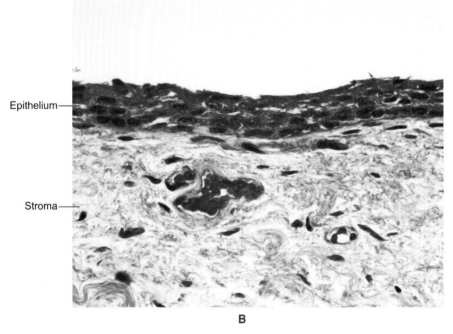

Epithelium

Stroma

B

Figures 2.2A and B. Normal vaginal mucosa: A. Mature vaginal squamous epithelium showing normal layering: basal layer, parabasal layer, intermediate layer, and superficial layers. Clearing of the cytoplasm in the upper layers is related to progressive accumulation of glycogen. B. Atrophic vaginal epithelium from a postmenopausal woman is thin and consists only of basal and parabasal cells.

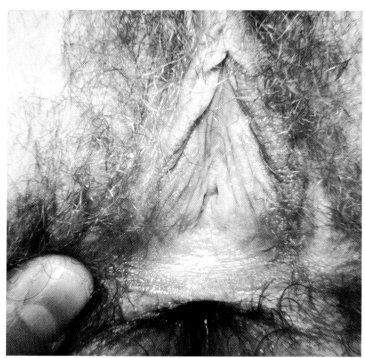

Figure 2.3. Vaginal agenesis: The vagina is absent and is replaced by a blind pouch. The vulva is otherwise normal.

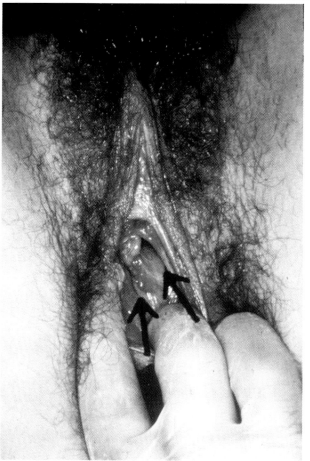

Figure 2.4. Duplication of the vagina: An incompletely formed longitudinal septum subdivides the vagina into two compartments (arrows).

the lesions are composed of glands lined by cells that have clear cytoplasm or resemble endocervical epithelium (Fig. 2.5).

2. *Endometriosis:* It refers to the presence of endometrial glands and stroma in the vaginal wall (Fig. 2.6). It is usually associated with episiotomy scars.

3. *Vaginal cysts:* It may originate from epithelial invaginations or from residual fetal structures. These cysts are microscopically different and are classified as follows:
   - *Epithelial inclusion cyst:* These cysts are lined by stratified squamous epithelium and are usually filled with keratin squames.
   - *Müllerian cyst:* These cysts are found in the upper vagina and are lined by tall columnar, mucin secreting cells.
   - *Mesonephric cyst (Gartner duct cyst):* These cysts are usually found in the lateral wall of the vagina. They are lined by low-cuboidal, clear cells that do not secrete mucin.

Benign Epithelial Tumors

1. *Squamous papilloma of the vagina:* It is an uncommon lesion that usually presents in the form of small wart-like mucosal protrusions. Clinically, it may be associated with a sense of burning or dyspareunia. Microscopically, it usually consists of a central fibrovascular core that is covered by squamous epithelium (Fig. 2.7). It must be distinguished from condyloma acuminatum.

2. *Condyloma acuminatum:* Also known as genital wart, condyloma acuminatum results from infection with non-oncogenic Human papillomaviruses. Clinically, such warts may appear exophytic (*papular* or *papillomatous*) or flat (*macular*). They are often multiple. Condylomata have diagnostic histologic and cytologic features (Fig. 2.8). These microscopic findings include thickening of the squamous epithelium (acanthosis), prominence of the surface keratin layer (*hyperkeratosis*), and elongation and branching of dermal connective tissue papillae (*papillomatosis*). The surface layers of the epithelium contain HPV infected cells (koilocytes) that have clear cytoplasm and irregularly shaped "raisin-like" nuclei. The most important features of condyloma acuminatum are listed in Box 2.1.

Box 2.1. Condyloma acuminatum
ETIOLOGY
•   Non-oncogenic HPV types 6 and 11
CLINICAL FEATURES
•   Single or multiple mucosal lesions
•   Warts, raised or flat
•   Located most often close to the introitus or in the vaginal fornices
HISTOPATHOLOGY
•   Acanthosis
•   Hyperkeratosis
•   Koilocytosis
•   Papillomatosis with vascularized connective tissue cores
HPV—Human papillomavirus

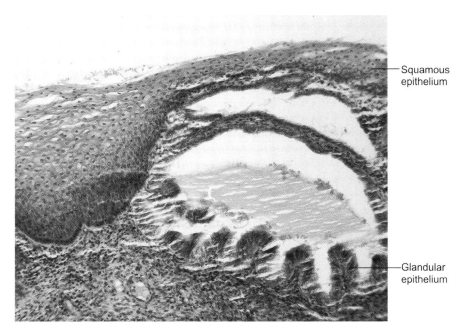

Squamous
epithelium

Glandular
epithelium

Figure 2.5. Vaginal adenosis: Mucin-secreting glands are present underneath the squamous epithelium of the vagina.

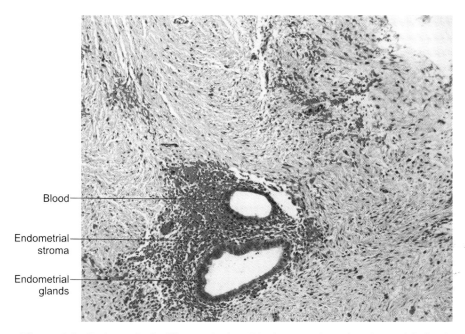

Blood

Endometrial
stroma

Endometrial
glands

Figure 2.6. Endometriosis: The vaginal wall lesion consists of endometrial glands and stroma. Extravasated blood is seen in the stroma.

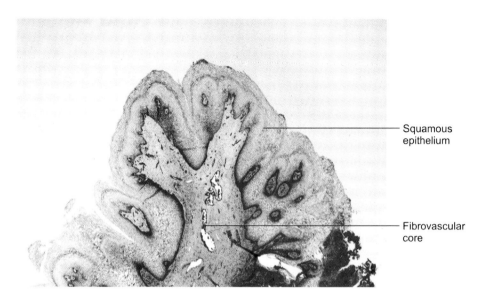

Squamous
epithelium

Fibrovascular
core

Figure 2.7. Squamous papilloma: This papillary structure has a central fibrovascular core covered with squamous epithelium. It lacks the complex branching of a typical condyloma acuminatum and it does not contain HPV-infected koilocytes.

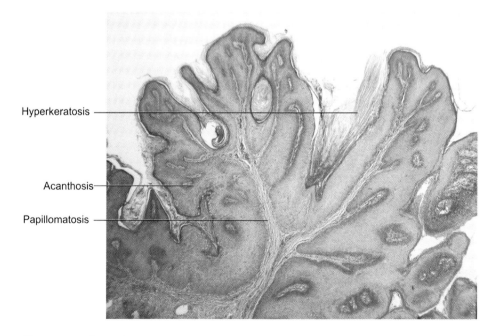

Hyperkeratosis

Acanthosis

Papillomatosis

Figure 2.8. Condyloma acuminatum: The lesion shows prominent papillomatosis and acanthosis. Koilocytes in the superficial layers are not clearly visible in this low-power microphotograph.

Vaginal Squamous Intraepithelial Neoplasia

Vaginal squamous intraepithelial neoplasia (VAIN) represents a premalignant alteration of the vaginal squamous epithelium related to HPV infection. Microscopically, VAIN has the same features as cervical intraepithelial neoplasia (CIN) and can be graded on scale from 1 to 3 as mild, moderate or severe (Box 2.2). VAIN 3 corresponds to carcinoma *in situ* (CIS).

In all forms of VAIN the biopsy shows characteristic microscopic changes. These changes vary from prominent koilocytosis and mildly disordered maturation in low-grade VAIN to complete disorganization of the entire epithelium in VAIN 3 (Fig. 2.9). Most VAINs regress even without treatment, but a small number of high-grade VAINs will progress to invasive carcinoma even after therapy.

Box 2.2. Vaginal squamous intraepithelial neoplasia (VAIN)
ETIOLOGY
HPV infection
-VAIN 1— low-risk HPV types
-VAIN 2 and VAIN 3— high-risk HPV types
(HPV 16 most common)
CLINICAL FEATURES
Asymptomatic
Abnormal cytologic findings*
Diagnosis made by a colposcopically directed biopsy
Usually involves the upper third of the vagina
PATHOLOGY
VAIN 1—koilocytosis, normal layering, and mildly disorganized basal layer
VAIN 2—disorganized layering in lower two-thirds of the squamous epithelium
VAIN 3—squamous dysplasia involving the full thickness of the epithelium+

+ *Note*: Overlying hyperkeratosis and parakeratosis are common in all forms of VAIN

Pearl: VAIN should be suspected if the cervical-vaginal smear contains dysplastic/atypical cells and the colposcopy reveals no cervical lesions

Vaginal Carcinomas

1. *Squamous cell carcinoma:* It is the most common malignant tumor of the vagina. Typically it is diagnosed in elderly women, and the mean age at the time of diagnosis is 60 years. It is mostly associated with persistent infection with high-risk HPV and it is usually preceded by high-grade VAIN. Previous radiation therapy for carcinoma of the cervix may be found in the history of some patients.

   The most common site of squamous cell carcinoma is the upper third of the vagina. Microscopically, these tumors have the typical features of either keratinizing or nonkeratinizing squamous cells carcinomas (Figs 2.10 and 2.11). Some tumors represent vaginal extension of primary or recurrent vulvar or cervical squamous cell carcinoma, from which they cannot be distinguished microscopically.

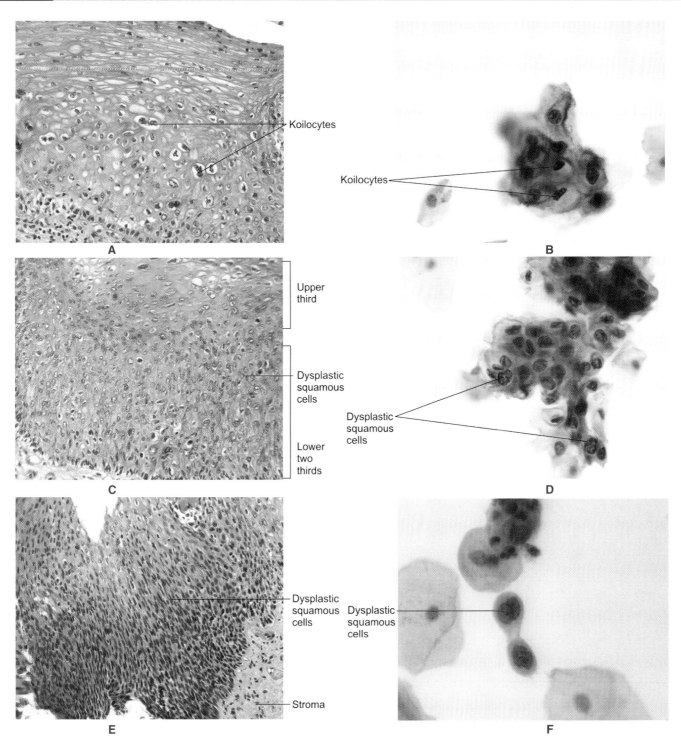

Figures 2.9A to F. Vaginal intraepithelial neoplasia (VAIN): A and B. VAIN 1. The epithelium is slightly thickened with prominent koilocytosis. The vaginal smear contains characteristic koilocytes with enlarged nuclei. The nuclear membranes of these cells are irregular and are surrounded by a clear perinuclear halo. C and D. VAIN 2. Disorganized squamous cells with enlarged nuclei, pleomorphism, and mitoses are evident in the lower two-thirds of the squamous epithelium. Vaginal smear shows a group of dysplastic squamous cells with a high nuclear-cytoplasmic ratio. E and F. VAIN 3. Dysplastic squamous cells involve the entire thickness of the squamous epithelium. Vaginal smear shows scattered highly dysplastic cells with enlarged hyperchromatic nuclei and scant cytoplasm.

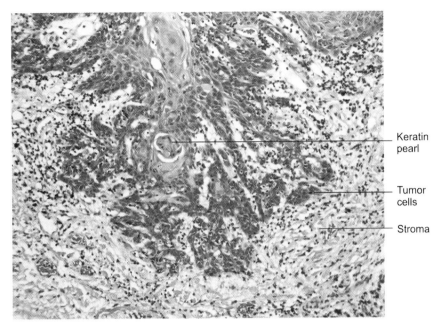

Keratin
pearl

Tumor
cells

Stroma

Figure 2.10. Squamous cell carcinoma: Tumor cells arising from the surface epithelium invade the superficial stroma. An eosinophilic keratin pearl can be seen in the middle of the field.

Box 2.3. Squamous cell carcinoma of the vagina

ETIOLOGY
- Persistent high-risk HPV infection*
- Prior pelvic irradiation
- Prior preinvasive or invasive cervical or vulvar cancer

CLINICAL FEATURES
- Maybe asymptomatic
- Painless bloody vaginal discharge
- Dysuria, postcoital bleeding, pelvic pain

PATHOLOGY
- Macroscopic: flat, exophytic, ulcerative, or annular
- Microscopic: squamous cell carcinoma

TREATMENT
- Radiation
- Radical excision for early stage disease

*Most common cause of neoplasia

The most important features of vaginal carcinoma are listed in Box 2.3.

2. *Verrucous carcinoma:* It is a very well differentiated variant of squamous cell carcinoma. Microscopically, it has a papillary growth pattern with pushing borders and bulbous pegs (Fig. 2.12). It invades into the stroma locally, but it is almost never associated with lymph node metastases.

3. *Clear cell adenocarcinoma:* It is a rare malignant tumor of young women. The mean age of patients at the time of diagnosis is 17 years. About two-thirds of cases are associated with *in utero* exposure to diethylstilbestrol (DES).

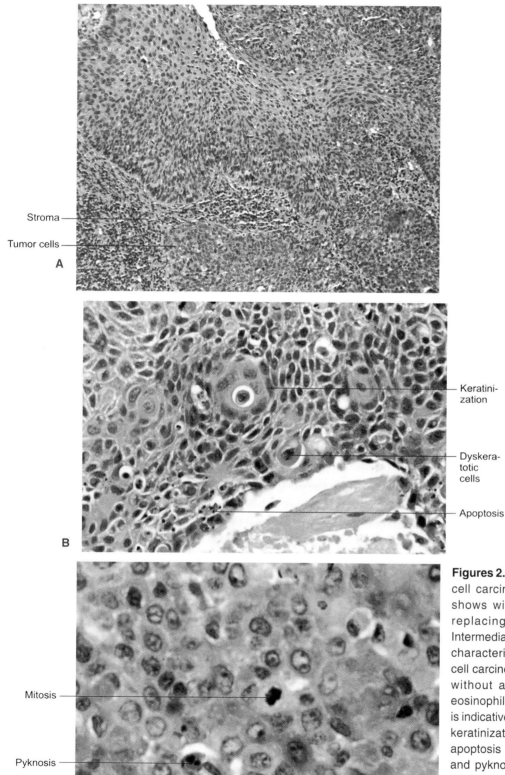

Stroma

Tumor cells

A

Keratini-zation

Dyskera-totic cells

Apoptosis

B

Mitosis

Pyknosis

C

Figures 2.11A to C. Invasive squamous cell carcinoma: A. Low power view shows wide strands of tumor cells replacing most of the stroma. B. Intermediate power view illustrating the characteristic features of squamous cell carcinoma. The cells are arranged without any distinct layering. The eosinophilic cytoplasm of some cells is indicative of keratinization. Single cell keratinization ("dyskeratosis"), foci of apoptosis recognized by karyorrhexis and pyknosis of tumor cell nuclei are also seen. C. High power view shows mitotic figures and pyknotic tumor cells undergoing apoptosis.

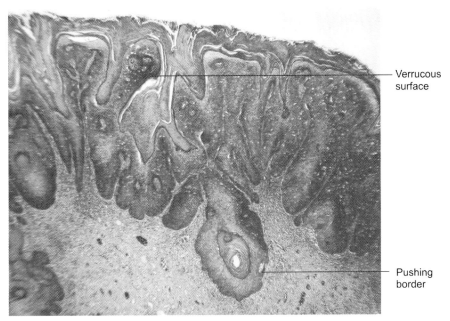

Verrucous surface

Pushing border

Figure 2.12. Verrucous carcinoma: The tumor is characterized by a proliferation of cytologically bland squamous cells forming bulbous masses. At the interface with the stroma the tumor nest have rounded contours accounting for the tumor's pushing, rather than obviously invasive margins.

Clear cell adenocarcinoma most commonly occurs in the upper part of the vagina and may also involve the cervix. Histologically it is composed of neoplastic glands and tubules lined by hobnailed clear cells filled with glycogen (Fig. 2.13). The most important features of clear cell carcinoma of the vagina are listed in Box 2.4.

Vaginal Mesenchymal Tumors and Tumor-like Lesions

1. *Fibroepithelial polyp:* It may not represent a true neoplasm, but rather a reactive/hyperplastic lesion. It is most often found in pregnant women. Histologically, it has a central fibrovascular core covered by normal squamous epithelium (Fig. 2.14). The stroma maybe edematous and contain thick-walled blood vessels. Large bizarre spindle-shaped connective tissue cells maybe present in the stroma of some lesions.

2. *Embryonal rhabdomyosarcoma (sarcoma botryoides):* It is a rare tumor of infancy and childhood. Even so it is the most common vaginal sarcoma. Almost all patients are less than 5 years of age. The tumor characteristically presents as a soft, polypoid and grape-like mass, often protruding from the vagina. The mucosa may be ulcerated and hemorrhagic (Fig. 2.15A). Microscopically, the tumor is composed of closely packed small blue

---

Box 2.4. Clear cell adenocarcinoma of the vagina

ETIOLOGY
- Prenatal exposure to DES (75%)

CLINICAL FEATURES
- A tumor of adolescent girls (mean age 17 years)
- Vaginal bleeding or discharge
- May be asymptomatic

PATHOLOGY
- Macroscopic: polypoid or nodular, less often flat or ulcerated
- Microscopic: adenocarcinoma composed of clear, hobnailed cells

TREATMENT
- Surgical resection
- Local radiotherapy

DES—Diethylstilbestrol

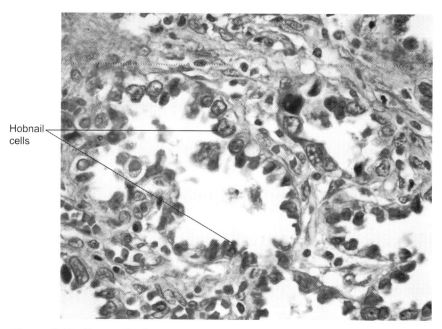

Hobnail cells

Figure 2.13. Clear cell adenocarcinoma: The tumor is composed of tubules lined by clear and hobnail cells.

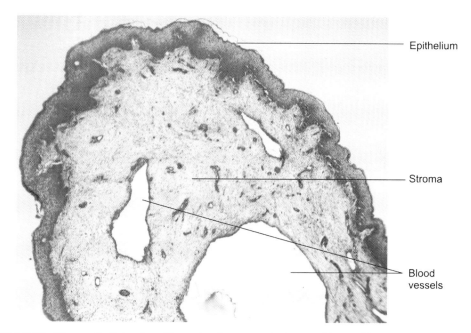

Epithelium

Stroma

Blood vessels

Figure 2.14. Fibroepithelial polyp: The polyp has a central core of loose fibrovascular stroma covered by normal squamous epithelium.

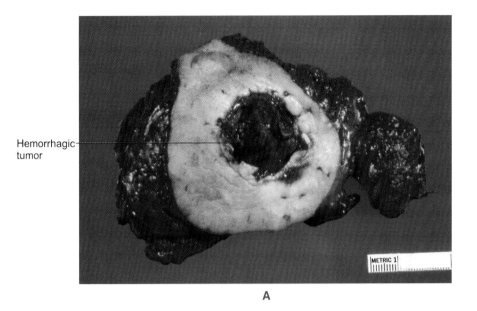

Hemorrhagic tumor

A

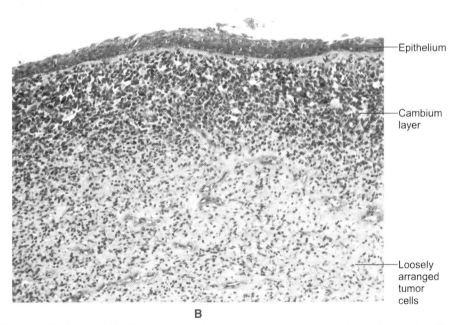

Epithelium

Cambium layer

Loosely arranged tumor cells

B

Figures 2.15A and B. Embryonal rhabdomyosarcoma (sarcoma botryoides): A. The tumor is located at the vaginal introitus of this radical vaginectomy specimen. It is ulcerated and appears hemorrhagic. B. Microscopically the tumor is composed of small spindle-shaped cells condensed into a subepithelial "cambium" layer. The surface of the polyp is covered with normal prepubertal squamous epithelium of the vagina.

cells with hyperchromatic nuclei and inconspicuous nucleoli (Fig. 2.15B). Scattered rhabdomyoblasts may be seen. Tumor cells are usually loosely arranged and the central part of the polypoid lesions is typically edematous. Underneath the normal squamous epithelium of the frond, the tumor cells are usually condensed forming a so-called *cambium* layer. Immunohistochemical staining with antibodies to muscle markers (e.g. *actin, desmin, myoglobin*) may be necessary to identify the neoplastic rhabdomyoblasts.

3

Uterine Cervix

NORMAL ANATOMY AND HISTOLOGY

The cervix is the most caudal cylindrical portion of the uterus, constituting up to 1/3rd of the entire uterine length. The endocervical canal connects the uterine corpus with the vagina (Fig. 3.1). The adult normal cervix measures 2.5 to 3.0 cm in diameter by 3.5 to 5.0 cm in length. It is divided into three parts: an upper, a supravaginal, and a lower vaginal portion. These portions are more or less of the same length.

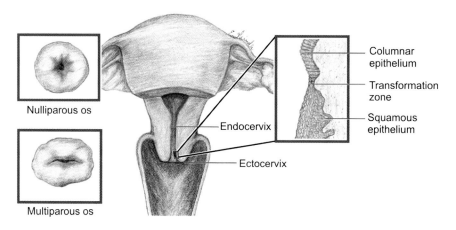

Figure 3.1. Normal cervix.

The aspects of normal anatomy and histology that are most important for the understanding of cervical pathology are as follows:

- *Portio vaginalis*, the part of the cervix protruding into the vagina, contains a centrally located opening known as the external *cervical os*. In nulliparous women it has a roughly circular shape, whereas in multiparous women is slit-like and divided into an anterior and a posterior lip (Fig. 3.1).
- *Ectocervix* is the external surface of the cervix covered by stratified non-keratinized squamous epithelium. This epithelium is continuous with the squamous epithelial lining of the vagina.
- *Endocervix* corresponds to the cervical canal allowing the communication between the vagina and the uterine cavity.

- *The squamous epithelium* of the ectocervix is histologically divided into three zones: basal, midzone, and superficial layers (Fig. 3.2A). The basal cells have relatively large nuclei surrounded by scant cytoplasm. As the cells mature toward the surface their nuclei become smaller and condensed, whereas the cytoplasm becomes more abundant and filled with glycogen. Under normal circumstances mitoses are seen only in the basal and parabasal cell layers.
  - Loss of normal layering and maturation of the ectocervical epithelium is typical of epithelial dysplasia and neoplasia and can be easily recognized in cervical biopsies.
  - Like the normal ectocervical epithelium carcinomas of the cervix are composed of squamous cells.
  - Normal squamous cells can be readily recognized in smears obtained by exfoliative cytology ("Pap smears") (Fig. 3.3A).
- The *endocervical canal* is lined by a single layer of tall columnar mucin producing *glandular epithelium*. The endocervical mucosa also lines the inside of endocervical glands, i.e. the branching invaginations of the cervical lumen (Fig. 3.2B). The endocervical glands are embedded within a prominent fibromuscular stroma.
  - Endocervical glandular epithelium is normally seen in properly prepared Pap smears (Fig. 3.3B).
  - Endocervical cancers originating from the glandular epithelium are adenocarcinomas.
- The border between the squamous ectocervical epithelium and the columnar endocervical epithelium is known as the *squamocolumnar junction* (SCJ). The anatomic location of the SCJ varies from one person to another and throughout life. It is also under hormonal influence.
  - The point of transition of the endocervical into squamous epithelium is known as the *transformation zone*. It is the site of origin of most cervical cancers and as such it must be sampled for cytologic smears.
  - The location of SCJ may be altered by *squamous metaplasia* that leads to replacement of the normal endocervical columnar epithelium by squamous epithelium.

OVERVIEW OF PATHOLOGY

The most important diseases of the cervix include the following entities:
- Inflammatory diseases and reactive lesions
- Neoplasms

Inflammatory Diseases and Reactive Lesions

This group of diseases includes nonspecific inflammation and various reactive lesions. The infections with human papillomavirus are discussed later together with neoplasms of the cervix to which they are intimately related.

1. *Cervicitis:* It is an inflammation of the cervix, which may involve the ectocervix, endocervix or both. It can be classified as acute and chronic depending on the type of inflammatory cells.
2. *Acute cervicitis:* It is an acute inflammation of the cervix characterized by an acute inflammatory infiltrate that can be associated with surface erosions or even deeper ulcerations (Fig. 3.4).
3. *Chronic inflammation of the endocervix:* It is a common finding in adult women. It is usually mild and of no clinical significance (Fig. 3.5). Intense chronic inflammatory changes, and certain microscopic findings could signify an association with specific infectious agents. The most important pathogens producing recognizable changes are as follows:

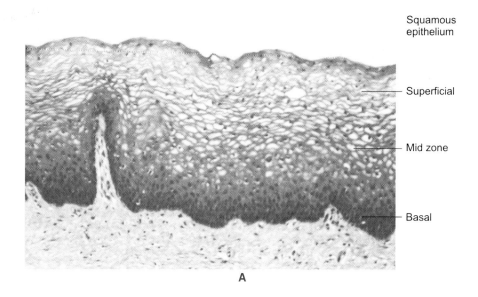

Squamous
epithelium

Superficial

Mid zone

Basal

A

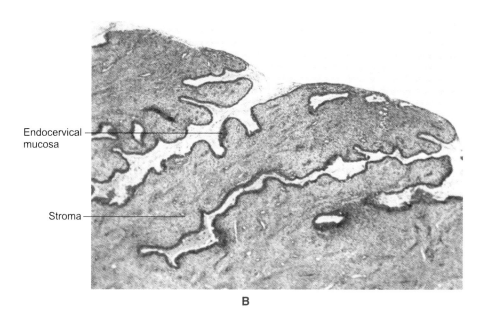

Endocervical
mucosa

Stroma

B

Figures 3.2A and B. Normal cervix: A. The ectocervix is lined by squamous epithelium. B. The endocervix is lined by columnar epithelium, which also lines the branching invaginations of the endocervical canal (endometrial glands).

- *Herpes simplex virus:* The infection is associated with epithelial ulceration resulting from the rupture of intraepithelial vesicles. Multinucleated epithelial cells with ground glass like intranuclear inclusions are typically seen in Pap smears (Fig. 3.6).
- *Chlamydia trachomatis*: The infection is often associated with an intense chronic inflammation and the formation of prominent lymphoid aggregates (*follicular cervicitis*).

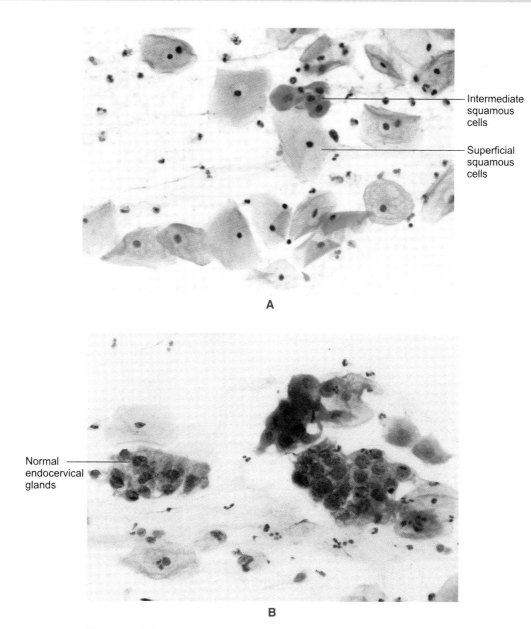

Intermediate squamous cells

Superficial squamous cells

A

Normal endocervical glands

B

Figures 3.3A and B. Normal cells obtained by exfoliative cytology of the cervix: A. The sample from the ectocervix contains a mixture of superficial and intermediate squamous cells. B. The endocervical sample contains columnar glandular cells with basally oriented nuclei (group to the left) or arranged in honeycomb pattern seen en-face (group to the right).

- *Trichomonas vaginalis:* The infection is associated with intraepithelial edema (*spongiosis*).
- *Cytomegalovirus:* The infection is accompanied by the appearance of large intranuclear and intracytoplasmic inclusions in the epithelial or endothelial cells.

4. *Endocervical polyps:* They are benign lesions that occur in up to 5 percent of adult women. They are composed of tissue protruding into the endocervical canal and even through the external os (Fig. 3.7). Microscopically,

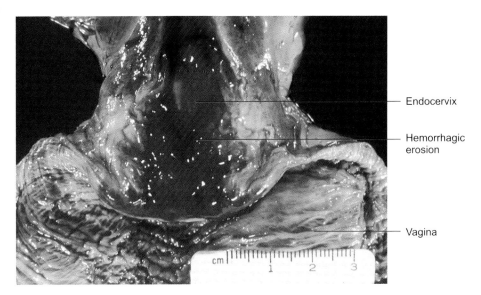

Endocervix

Hemorrhagic
erosion

Vagina

Figure 3.4. Cervical erosions: A hemorrhagic ulceration is seen in the
endocervical canal and extending almost to the vaginal surface of the ectocervix.

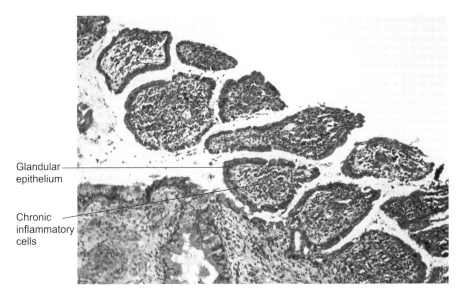

Glandular
epithelium

Chronic
inflammatory
cells

Figure 3.5. Chronic papillary cervicitis: Numerous papillae of the
endocervical mucosa are infiltrated by an intense chronic inflammatory
infiltrate.

polyps are composed of a dense fibrous stroma containing thick-walled vessels and glands (Fig. 3.8). On their external surface polyps are covered by normal endocervical epithelium. Those close to the external cervical os may be covered with squamous epithelium. Clinically, most of them are asymptomatic. Polyps protruding through the external os may cause irregular vaginal spotting, pain, and inflammation. The treatment is based on surgical removal.

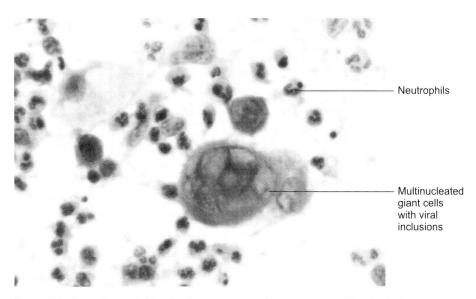

Neutrophils

Multinucleated
giant cells
with viral
inclusions

Figure 3.6. Herpetic cervicitis: The Pap smear contains classic multinucleated giant cells in a background of acute inflammation. The multiple nuclei contain intranuclear inclusions.

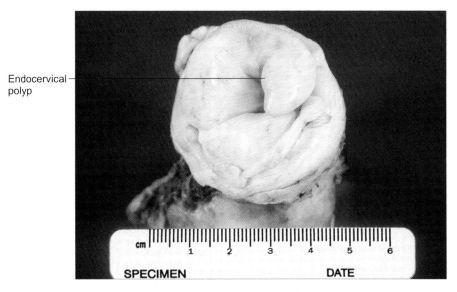

Endocervical
polyp

Figure 3.7. Endocervical polyp protruding through the external os.

Cervical Intraepithelial Neoplasia

Cervical intraepithelial neoplasia (CIN) also known as *squamous intraepithelial lesions (SIL)* is characterized by disordered growth and maturation of the squamous epithelium of the ectocervix. It is usually associated with human papillomavirus (HPV) infection. The complex interaction between various subtypes of HPV can be influenced by a variety of risk factors, which ultimately determine whether the lesion will have a self-limited course or progress to invasive carcinoma (Box 3.1).

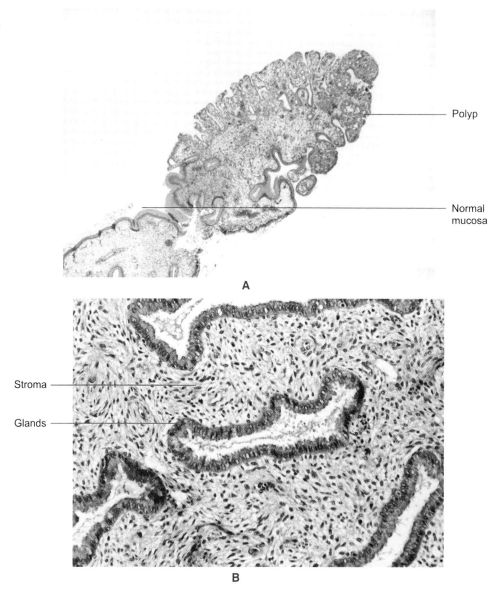

Polyp

Normal mucosa

A

Stroma

Glands

B

Figures 3.8A and B. Endocervical polyp: A. The oval-shaped polyp is attached to the normal cervical mucosa (left lower corner). B. At higher magnification the polyp appears composed of fibrous vascularized stroma and normal cervical glands.

Box 3.1. Risk factors for cervical intraepithelial neoplasia (CIN)

HPV infection *

Early age at first coitus

Multiple sexual partners

Increased parity

Other genital infections

Pearl: HPV are classified as low risk and high risk. The most common low risk HPV types are 6 and 11. High-risk types of HPV associated with cancer are 16, 18, 31, and 33.

According to the extent of dysplasia CIN can be graded as mild, moderate or severe or alternatively labeled as CIN 1, CIN 2 and CIN 3. According to The Bethesda system (TBS) these lesions are called *squamous intraepithelial lesions* (SIL) and graded as low grade or high grade. The comparison of these systems is given in Box 3.2.

The microscopic and cytologic features of various forms of CIN are listed in Boxes 3.3 to 3.5 and illustrated in Figures 3.9 to 3.15.

Papanicolaou smear ("Pap smear") is widely used as a screening test for cervical intraepithelial neoplasia and cancer. At the present time the TBS is most commonly used for reporting cervical/ vaginal cytologic diagnoses of Pap smears.

The Pap smear findings reported according to the TBS classification, as formulated in 2001 are classified as squamous cell changes (Box 3.6) or glandular change (Box 3.7). These cytologic findings correlated with the corresponding microscopic pathologic changes seen in cervical biopsies are shown in Figures 3.9 to 3.15.

Invasive Neoplasia of the Cervix

Two malignant neoplasms, squamous cell carcinoma and adenocarcinoma account for more than 98% of all cervical malignancies.

1. *Squamous cell carcinoma:* It is the most common form of malignancy of the cervix. HPV has been detected in up to 90% of squamous carcinoma indicating that this virus plays an important pathogenetic role. In most instances invasive carcinoma is preceded by CIN, and accordingly the risk factors for cervical squamous cell carcinoma are the same as for CIN. Other salient features about squamous cell carcinoma are listed in Box 3.8. The principal macroscopic and microscopic aspects of cervical squamous cells carcinoma are summarized in Boxes 3.9 and 3.10 and illustrated in Figures 3.16 to 3.23.

Box 3.2. Comparison of three systems for grading and reporting of cervical intraepithelial neoplasia

Descriptive terms	Cervical intraepithelial neoplasia (CIN)	The Bethesda system (TBS)
Mild squamous dysplasia	CIN 1	Low grade SIL
HPV related changes	CIN 1	Low grade SIL
Moderate squamous dysplasia	CIN 2	High grade SIL
Severe squamous dysplasia	CIN 3	High grade SIL
Carcinoma *in situ*	CIN 3	High grade SIL

SIL—squamous intraepithelial lesion

Box 3.3. Histopathology of mild squamous dysplasia (CIN 1)

- Surface maturation of epithelium well preserved
- Changes limited to the lower third of the epithelium
  - Nuclear pleomorphism, mild
  - Nuclear hyperchromasia, mild to moderate
  - Mitoses, rare
  - Koilocytosis, usually present

Box 3.4. Histopathology of moderate squamous dysplasia (CIN 2)

- Surface maturation of epithelium still evident
- Changes involve one half or two-third of the epithelium
  - Nuclear pleomorphism, prominent
  - Nuclear hyperchromasia, prominent
  - Mitoses, limited to lower two-third of the epithelium
  - Abnormal mitoses maybe present
  - Koilocytosis, usually present

Box 3.5. Histopathology of severe squamous dysplasia (CIN 3)

- No evidence of surface maturation*
- Changes involve the entire thickness of the epithelium
  - High nuclear-cytoplasmic ratio
  - Nuclear hyperchromasia, marked
  - Nucleoli prominent and easily identified
  - Mitoses in all layers, often abnormal

Pearls: The epithelium lacks any layering and if were turned upside down it would look the same as when normally positioned.

A surface parakeratotic layer is seen in many cases.

Box 3.6. Reporting of squamous cell changes in cytologic smears

- Atypical squamous cells of undetermined significance (ASCUS)
- Atypical squamous cells of undetermined significance—cannot exclude HGSIL
- Low-grade squamous intraepithelial lesion (LGSIL)
  - Encompassing HPV changes and/or CIN 1 (mild dysplasia).
- High-grade squamous intraepithelial lesion (HGSIL)
  - Encompassing: CIN 2 (moderate dysplasia) CIN 3 (severe dysplasia and carcinoma in situ) with features suggestive of invasion, if invasion is suspected
- Squamous cell carcinoma

Box 3.7. Reporting of glandular cell changes in cytologic smears

- Atypical glandular cells of undetermined significance (AGUS) (endocervical/endometrial/glandular cells)
- Atypical glandular/endocervical cells, favor neoplastic
- Endocervical adenocarcinoma in situ
- Adenocarcinoma (endocervical/endometrial/extrauterine adenocarcinoma or adenocarcinoma not otherwise specified)

Box 3.9. Histopathology of cervical squamous cell carcinoma

- Ectropion-like (not obvious on naked eye examination)
- Exophytic*
  - Polypoid
- Endophytic
  - Ulcerated
  - Mostly endocervical producing a "barrel shaped" cervix
- Mixed exophytic and endophytic

*Pearl: Most tumors are exophytic

Box 3.8. Squamous cell carcinoma of the cervix

EPIDEMIOLOGY
- 13,000 new cases per year diagnosed in the US*
- 7,000 deaths per year in the US
- Preceded by CIN 2 or CIN 3 in most cases
- Mean age at diagnosis is 55 years

RISK FACTORS
- HPV infection with types 16,18, 31, 33, 35, 39
- Early age at first coitus
- Multiple sexual partners
- Increased parity
- Other genital infections

CLINICAL FEATURES
- Asymptomatic (most often)
- Bleeding
- Dyspareunia

THERAPY
- Surgery and radiation therapy

*Note: The incidence of cervical squamous cells carcinoma has decreased in the US over the last 50 years, mostly due to effective cytologic screening programs

Box 3.10. Microscopic subtypes of cervical invasive squamous cell carcinoma

- Keratinizing*
- Nonkeratinizing
- Rare variants
  - Warty (condylomatous)
  - Verrucous
  - Papillary squamous
  - Lymphoepithelioma-like
- Microinvasive carcinoma

*Pearl: Keratinizing squamous cell carcinoma is the most common form of cervical carcinoma

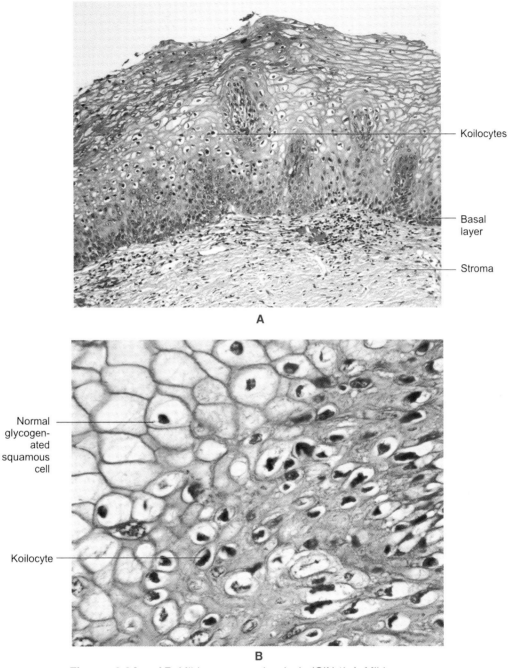

Figures 3.9A and B. Mild squamous dysplasia (CIN 1): A. Mild squamous dysplasia and human papillomavirus related changes involve the lower third of the epithelium whereas the superficial cells show normal layering. B. Koilocytes have irregularly shaped nuclei and clear cytoplasm.

The incidence of this tumor in many other countries is higher than in the USA.

2. *Microinvasive squamous cell carcinoma* (FIGO stage Ia1): It is a subset of cervical cancer diagnosed during the early stages of transition between CIN 3 to overtly invasive carcinoma (Fig. 3.21). The criteria for diagnosing microinvasive squamous cell carcinoma are listed in Box 3.11.

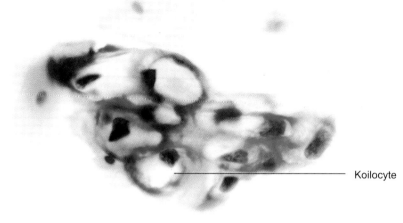

Koilocyte

Figure 3.10. Low-grade squamous intraepithelial lesion (LGSIL). The Pap smear contains koilocytes. These cells have hyperchromatic nuclei lacking internal details ("smudging of chromatin"), and show characteristic cytoplasmic vacuolization ("perinuclear halo").

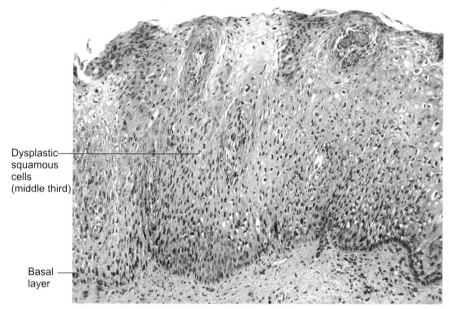

Dysplastic squamous cells (middle third)

Basal layer

Figure 3.11. Moderate squamous dysplasia (CIN 2): A. Dysplasia involves more than one half of the entire thickness of the epithelium. Occasional atypical mitoses are noted.

**Box 3.11. Cervical microinvasive squamous cell carcinoma—
histopathology (according to FIGO)**

- Tumor diagnosed microscopically but was not identifiable on gross examination
- Intraepithelial squamous cell carcinoma (CIN 3) present on the surface
- Foci of invasion of the underlying stroma present
    - Tumor depth: less than 3 mm as measured from the closest basal layer of the overlying epithelium to the deepest point of invasion
    - Tumor diameter, i.e. horizontal spread: less than 7 mm
    - Angiolymphatic invasion not identified

FIGO—International Federation of Gynecologists and Obstetricians

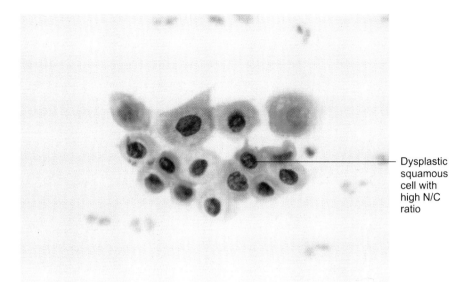

Figure 3.12. High-grade squamous intraepithelial lesions (HGSIL): Pap smear shows dysplastic squamous cells. These cells have a high nuclear/cytoplasmic ratio as compared to LGSIL cells.

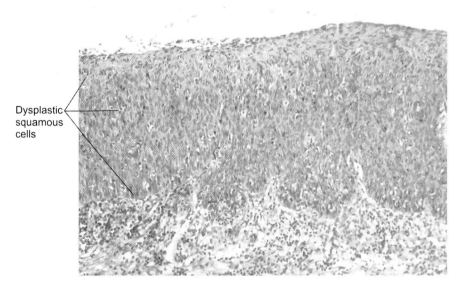

Figure 3.13. Severe squamous dysplasia (CIN 3): The epithelium shows no signs of maturation and the dysplastic cells are seen in all layers.

Cervical squamous cell carcinomas metastasize to regional lymph nodes, which must be dissected during surgery. Metastases are identified histologically in lymph nodes on intraoperative frozen sections or in permanent sections prepared from paraffin embedded lymph nodes (Fig. 3.22).

Exfoliative cytology plays an important role in early detection of cervical carcinoma. Characteristic cytologic features of cervical squamous cell carcinoma as seen in Pap smears are illustrated in Figure 3.23.

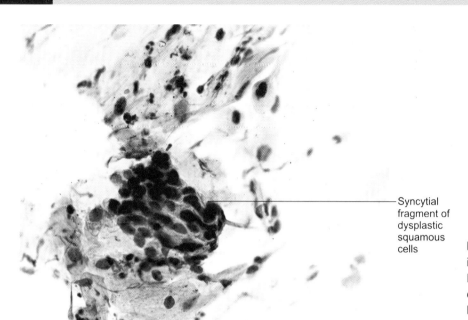

Syncytial fragment of dysplastic squamous cells

Figure 3.14. High-grade squamous intraepithelial lesions (HGSIL): The Pap smear shows a syncytial group of dysplastic squamous cells with hyperchromatic nuclei and high nuclear to cytoplasmic ratio.

3. *Endocervical adenocarcinoma:* It accounts for 20% of all cervical carcinomas, but its incidence is rising. It is related to HPV infection with risk types of virus (Box 3.12).

The clinical features of endocervical carcinoma are summarized in Box 3.13. Because of the difficulties in clinically diagnosing endocervical carcinoma, Pap smears provide the only hope for early diagnosis, *i.e.* early in the course of the disease when these tumors are still surgically curable.

The neoplasm presents with typical macroscopic and microscopic changes reflecting the progression from early intraepithelial neoplasia to invasive cancer (Box 3.14). It should be noticed, nevertheless, that no obvious macroscopic changes are found in up to 20% of all women showing diagnostic cytologic abnormalities in Pap smears.

Endocervical adenocarcinoma *in situ* is diagnosed microscopically using the criteria listed in Box 3.15 and illustrated in Figure 3.24. The diagnosis can be made cytologically in Pap smears as well (Fig. 3.25).

Invasive endocervical adenocarcinoma may present in several histopathologic forms (Box 3.16). Mucinous and endometrioid adenocarcinomas account for over 90% of all malignant tumors of endocervix. Typical histopathologic and cytologic features of these tumors are illustrated in Figures 3.26 and 3.27.

Box 3.12. Epidemiology of endocervical adenocarcinoma

- 10-20% of all cervical cancers
- Incidence is rising
- HIV infection with types 16 and 18 most common
- Peak age at diagnosis is 55 years

Box 3.13. Clinical features of cervical adenocarcinoma

- Almost all preinvasive tumors are asymptomatic* and not visible by colposcopy
- 20% of invasive tumors are asymptomatic* and many are invisible during colposcopy
- Symptoms
  - Vaginal discharge
  - Abnormal vaginal bleeding
  - Pain
  - Post-coital bleeding
- Symptoms in advanced cases
  - Pelvic mass
  - Invasion of pelvic organs
  - Distant metastases

Pearl: Abnormal Pap smear may be the only diagnostic finding

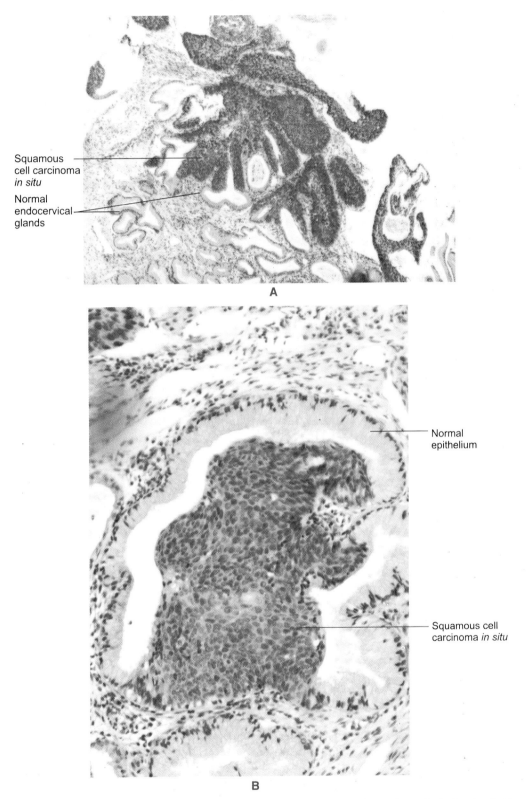

Squamous
cell carcinoma
in situ

Normal
endocervical
glands

A

Normal
epithelium

Squamous cell
carcinoma *in situ*

B

Figures 3.15A and B. Squamous cell carcinoma *in situ* (CIN 3): Extending into the endocervical glands. A. Hyperchromatic dysplastic squamous cells occupy some of the endocervical glands. B. Higher magnification view of CIN 3 partially replacing the normal endocervical glandular epithelium.

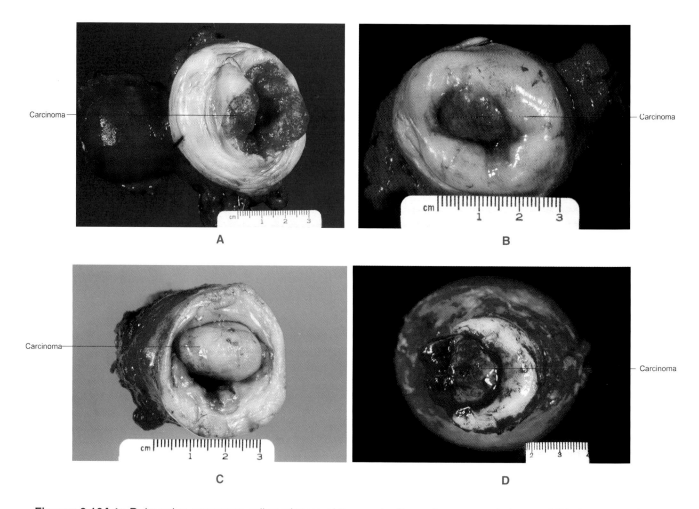

Carcinoma

Carcinoma

A

B

Carcinoma

Carcinoma

C

D

Figures 3.16A to D. Invasive squamous cell carcinoma of the cervix: Several macroscopic forms of this tumor are shown: A. Exophytic, B. Mostly endocervical, C. Polypoid, and D. Mixed exophytic and ulcerated.

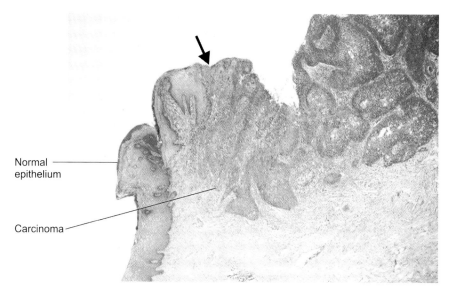

Normal epithelium

Carcinoma

Figure 3.17. Invasive squamous cell carcinoma of the cervix: The arrow points to the transition of the normal epithelium (to the left) into carcinoma (to the right).

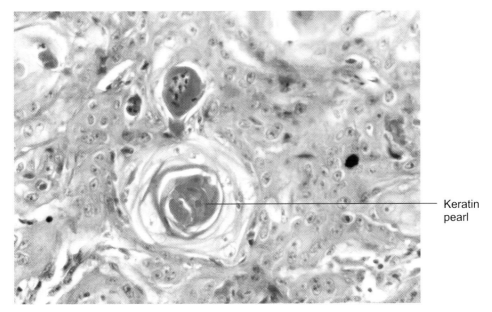

Keratin
pearl

Figure 3.18. Invasive squamous cell carcinoma of the cervix: There are prominent keratin pearls indicative of keratinization.

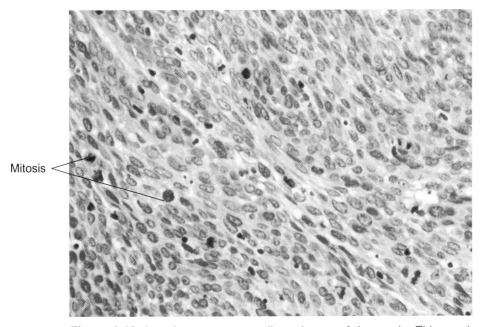

Mitosis

Figure 3.19. Invasive squamous cell carcinoma of the cervix: This poorly differentiated non-keratinizing squamous cell carcinoma is composed of small cells forming dense sheets. There are numerous mitoses but there is no keratinization.

During the histologic examination the pathologists are required to grade the tumors according to established criteria (Box 3.17). The depth of tumor invasion, which is important for the staging of carcinoma should be

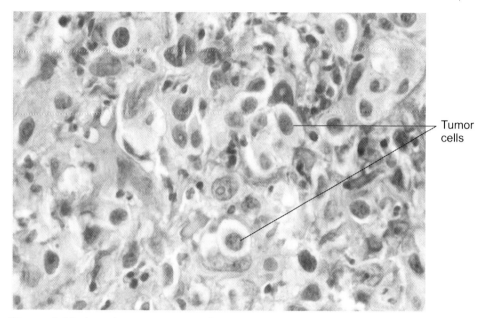

Tumor
cells

Figure 3.20. Invasive squamous cell carcinoma of the cervix: This poorly differentiated non-keratinizing squamous cell carcinoma is composed of pleomorphic large cells. There is no keratinization. Small inflammatory cells are seen between the tumor cells.

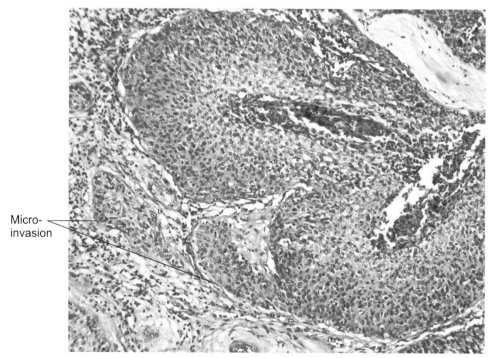

Micro-
invasion

Figure 3.21. Microinvasive squamous cell carcinoma of the cervix: Tongues of malignant squamous epithelium extend into the stroma. Note the stromal inflammatory response that is almost always present at the site of early invasion.

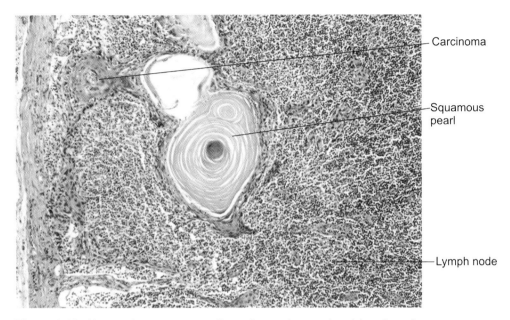

Figure 3.22. Metastatic squamous cell carcinoma in a regional lymph node. The lymph node contains tumor cells forming focally a large keratin pearl.

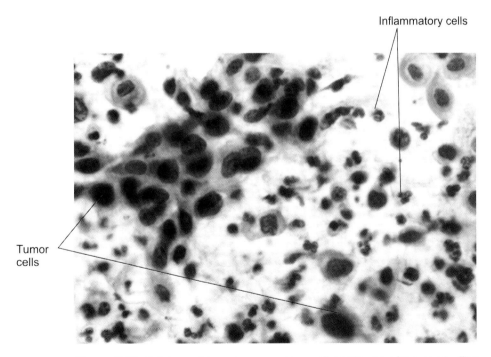

Figure 3.23. Cytology of invasive squamous cell carcinoma of the cervix. The smear contains groups and individual discohesive highly anaplastic malignant cells. The cells show marked pleomorphism and nuclear hyperchromasia.

Box 3.14. Macroscopic pathology of endocervical adenocarcinoma

- No macroscopic changes (20%)
  - Preinvasive adenocarcinoma (*in situ*)
  - Early invasive adenocarcinoma
- Exophytic
  - Polypoid lesions (most common)
  - Papillary
  - Nodular
- Endophytic
  - Ulcerated

Box 3.16. Microscopic subtypes of endocervical adenocarcinoma

- Mucinous adenocarcinoma
  - Endocervical subtype
  - Intestinal subtype
- Endometrioid adenocarcinoma
- Less common types:
  - Minimal deviation adenocarcinoma
  - Villoglandular adenocarcinoma
  - Clear cell adenocarcinoma
  - Serous adenocarcinoma

Box 3.15. Histopathology of endocervical adenocarcinoma *in situ*

- Normal glandular cells replaced by neoplastic cells*
- Cells show nuclear hyperchromasia, high nuclear to cytoplasmic ratio, abundant mitotic activity and individual cell necrosis
- No stromal invasion

---

* Microscopic changes may be limited to a single focus or multifocal

---

Box 3.17. Grading of endocervical adenocarcinoma

- Well differentiated, more than 50% glands
- Moderately differentiated, 10 to 50% glands
- Poorly differentiated, less than 10% glands

Adenocarcinoma *in situ*

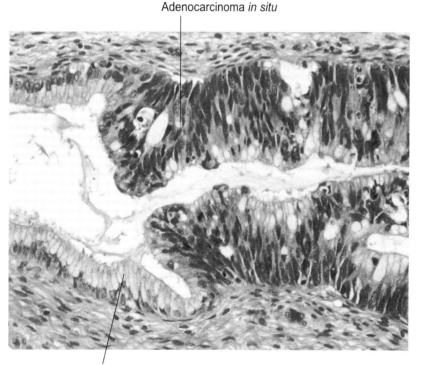

Normal endocervical glands

Figure 3.24. Adenocarcinoma *in situ* of the endocervix: There is a sharp border between the hyperchromatic neoplastic cells on the right and the normal mucinous cells on the left inside the same endocervical gland.

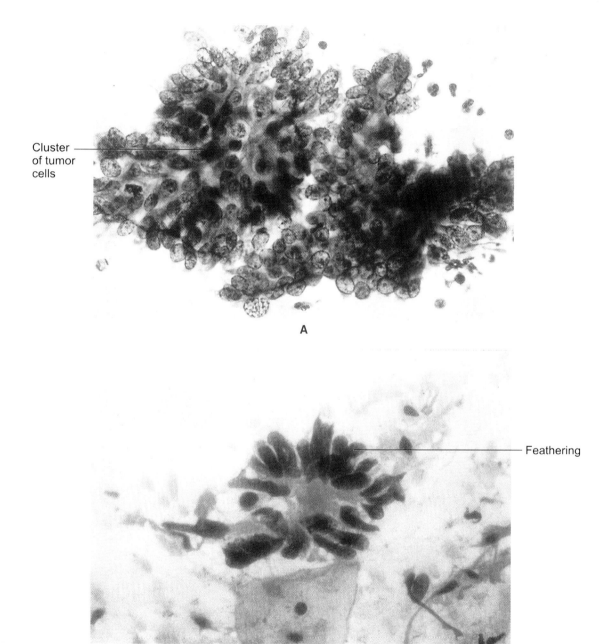

Cluster of tumor cells

Feathering

Figures 3.25A and B. Adenocarcinoma *in situ* of the endocervix: A. The malignant cells show marked nuclear overlapping and are clustered into crowded groups. B. The tumor cell nuclei arranged in a palisading manner protrude from the periphery of the cell cluster. This typical finding is known as "feathering".

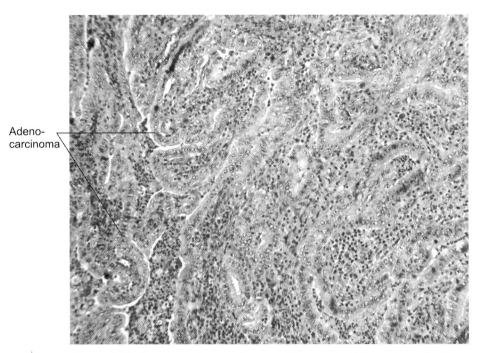

Adeno-
carcinoma

Figure 3.26. Invasive adenocarcinoma of the cervix: This endocervical type adenocarcinoma is composed of tall columnar cells interlacing through a background of inflammatory cells.

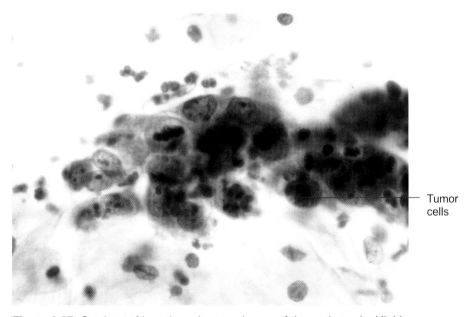

Tumor
cells

Figure 3.27. Cytology of invasive adenocarcinoma of the endocervix. Highly pleomorphic large tumor cells have prominent nucleoli and show irregular clumping of the chromatin.

expressed in percent involvement of the wall. It is determined by measuring the thickness of the tumor from the surface of the overlying epithelium to the deepest point of invasion.

Endocervical adenocarcinomas metastasize to regional lymph nodes like the cervical squamous cell carcinoma. The prognosis of cervical adenocarcinomas depends on the tumor stage. Tumor grade has also prognostic significance. When compared stage by stage the prognosis of endocervical adenocarcinoma is similar to the prognosis of squamous cell carcinoma of the cervix, or only slightly worse.

4

Uterine Corpus

NORMAL ANATOMY AND HISTOLOGY

The uterus is a pear-shaped hollow organ located between the rectum posteriorly and urinary bladder anteriorly. The adult nulliparous uterus weighs 40 to 100 gm and measures 8 cm in length, 5 cm in width and 2.5 cm in thickness. It is divided into the cervix (discussed in Chapter 3) and the corpus. The corpus uteri is divided into fundus, corpus and isthmus (Fig. 4.1). The two lateral corners of the fundus in connection with the intramural portion of the fallopian tubes insertion are referred to as the cornua. The isthmus or lower uterine segment refers to the portion that connects the corpus with cervix. The uterus is supported by the round and utero-ovarian ligaments.

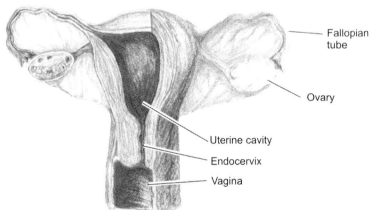

Figure 4.1. Normal uterus, cervix and bilateral fallopian tubes and ovaries.

The uterine cavity is lined by endometrium and surrounded by a thick smooth muscle layer called myometrium. The serosa is covered by pelvic peritoneum that extends to the point of peritoneal reflection which is lower in the posterior than the anterior aspect.

The important aspects of endometrium and myometrium histology that are most important for the understanding of pathology of uterine corpus are as follows:

• The *endometrium* is composed of glands and stroma (Fig. 4.2).

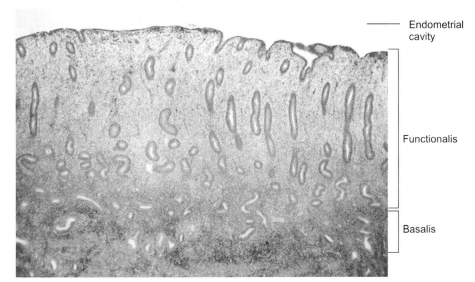

Figure 4.2. Normal endometrium: The top two-third is the functionalis layer that undergoes cyclic changes during reproductive years. The lower one-third is the basalis layer that has more dense stroma. There is no sharp demarcation between the functionalis layer and the basalis layer and between the basalis layer and the myometrium.

- Tumor can arise from the glandular component (as adenocarcinomas), stromal component (as endometrial stromal sarcomas), or both components (as malignant mixed mullerian tumors).

• The *functionalis layer,* comprising the upper two-third of the endometrial mucosa, undergoes cyclic changes during reproductive ages. The *basalis layer*, corresponding to the lower third, is responsible for the regeneration of the endometrium after menstruation. It does not change during the menstrual cycle.

• The normal endometrium undergoes *cyclic changes* during the menstrual cycle. The endometrial biopsy can be used to determine whether the endometrium is in the proliferative (Fig. 4.3) or secretory phase (Fig. 4.4). The daily morphologic changes in the *proliferative phase* are not sufficiently characteristic for accurate dating; however, the daily alterations in the *secretory phase* are distinct enough to permit accurate dating of the secretory phase of the menstrual cycle. The morphologic features of the proliferative and secretory phase endometrium are summarized in the Boxes 4.1 and 4.2.

Box 4.1. Microscopic features of normal proliferative endometrium

PROLIFERATIVE PHASE
- Early (4th-7th day)—short straight glands; compact stroma with some mitotic activity
- Mid (8th-10th day)—longer coiled glands with columnar surface epithelium; stromal edema, numerous mitosis, naked nuclei
- Late (11th-14th day)—tortuous glands with pseudostratified epithelium and mitotic activity; moderately dense stroma

INTERVAL PHASE (14th-15th day)—no notable changes for 36-48 hours after ovulation

Box 4.2. Microscopic features of secretory phase endometrium

EARLY SECRETORY (16th–20th day, glandular changes predominate)

- 16th day – subnuclear vacuoles, while the stroma still shows features of proliferative phase
- 17th day – orderly vacuolation with rows of nuclei lined up and large vacuoles below
- 18th day – vacuoles decrease in size, early secretions in lumen, nuclei approach base of cell
- 19th day – few vacuoles, intraluminal secretions, no pseudostratification, no mitoses
- 20th day – intraluminal secretions abundant.

MID TO LATE SECRETORY (21st-27th day, stromal changes predominate, secretory exhaustion)

- 21st day – secretory material in the lumen, abrupt marked stromal edema
- 22nd day –secretory material in the lumen, peak of stromal edema, naked nuclei
- 23rd day – prominent spiral arteries; periarteriolar predecidual change
- 24th day – rugged outline of glands, periarteriolar predecidual change; stromal mitoses recur
- 25th day – glands contain inspissated material; predecidual change under surface epithelium; increased stromal granular lymphocytes
- 26th day – confluent predecidual change, neutrophil influx begins
- 27th day – confluent sheets of decidua, more prominent granular lymphocytes, focal necrosis with leukocytes
- 28th day – prominent necrosis, hemorrhage and leukocytes.

- Inadequate proliferative phase or inadequate secretory phase may lead to dysfunctional bleeding.
- Exogenous administration of hormones affect the morphology of endometrium.

- If pregnancy occurs, the secretory-phase endometrium undergoes further morphologic development (reappearance of glandular secretion, stromal edema and vascular congestion, and predecidual reaction) and is referred to as *gestational endometrium*.
  - An exaggerated change in the gestational glands produces the *Arias-Stella reaction* characterized by prominent intraluminal epithelial projections composed of large cells with clear or eosinophilic cytoplasm, large hyperchromatic nuclei and irregular nuclear membranes (Fig. 4.5). The Arias-Stella reaction is usually focal, when extensive, it should not be confused with malignancy. These changes can also occur in the cervix, endometriosis, and adenomyosis.
- *Atrophic or inactive endometrium* is thin (less than 0.5 mm in thickness). Glands are few and resemble those in mid proliferative-phase with pseudostratified nuclei and lacking mitoses. Some glands are oriented parallel to the surface. The stroma is uniformly dense and often collagenized and resembles the stroma of lower uterine segment (Fig. 4.6).
- *Myometrium* is composed of smooth muscle cells arranged into bundles surrounded by fibrous tissue containing blood vessels. Smooth muscle cells of the myometrium have estrogen receptors.
  - Leiomyomas of the uterus are extremely common during the women's reproductive life. After menopause leiomyomas shrink in size, lose estrogen sensitive smooth muscle cells and transform into fibroids, i.e. tumors composed predominantly of fibroblastic connective tissue.

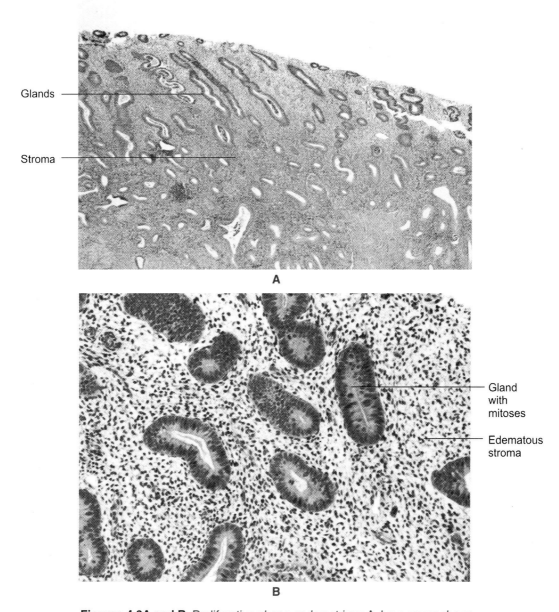

Figures 4.3A and B. Proliferative phase endometrium: A. Low-power shows long coiled glands with dense and focally edematous stroma. B. High-power view illustrating pseudostratified epithelium with mitoses and stroma edema, representing mid-proliferative phase.

OVERVIEW OF PATHOLOGY

The most important diseases of the uterine corpus are classified as follows:

- Infectious diseases
- Hormonally-induced changes
- Neoplasms

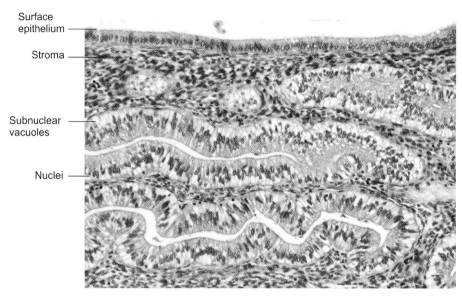

Surface epithelium

Stroma

Subnuclear vacuoles

Nuclei

Figure 4.4. Secretory phase endometrium: Early secretory phase endometrium contains glands with subnuclear vacuoles. The nuclei are lined up in a row just above the vacuoles in the midportion of the cells (day 17).

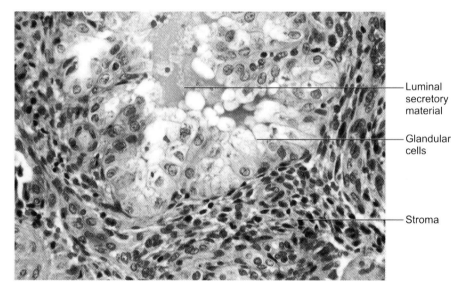

Luminal secretory material

Glandular cells

Stroma

Figure 4.5. Gestational endometrium: The glands are hyperplastic with intraluminal projections and secretions. The glandular cells are large with abundant clear cytoplasm and enlarged nuclei (*Arias-Stella reaction*).

Infectious Diseases

Endometritis

Endometritis is an inflammation of the endometrium, that may occur in an isolated form or as part of the pelvic inflammatory disease (PID). It can be classified as acute or chronic based on the type of inflammatory cells in the

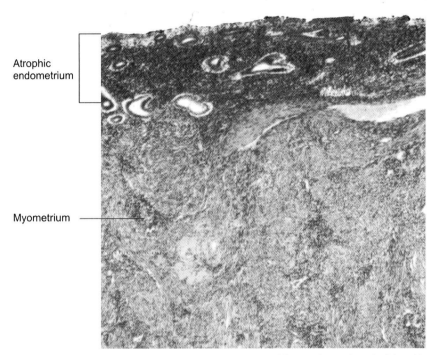

Atrophic
endometrium

Myometrium

Figure 4.6. Atrophic endometrium: The endometrium is thin with dense and collagenized stroma and few glands parallel to the surface.

endometrium; these terms do not necessarily correspond with the actual duration of the process. Sometimes, a specific etiologic agent can be identified whereas in others the causes are never identified.

1. *Acute endometritis:* It is typically related to ascending infection. Most often it is found after termination of pregnancy, as in the postpartum period or after spontaneous and induced abortion. It also occurs following any type of intrauterine instrumentation or surgery. Histologically, it is characterized by infiltration of the endometrium with polymorphonuclear leukocytes destroying and filling endometrial glands and forming microabscesses in the stroma (Fig. 4.7). It should be noted that normal premenstrual endometrial glands (on days 26 to 28) may contain neutrophils and debris in the lumen; these changes should not be misinterpreted as acute endometritis.

2. *Chronic endometritis:* Traditionally it has been classified as *non-specific*, when no specific microorganisms are identified, or *specific* when a particular pathogen is identified. For example chronic endometritis associated with *Chlamydia trachomatis*, or *Mycoplasma hominis* may be identified by culture of endometrial biopsy tissue.

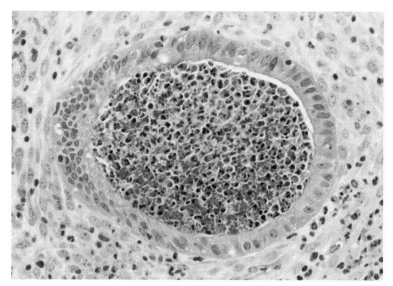

Figure 4.7. Acute endometritis: An endometrial gland is filled with neutrophils forming a microabscess.

Tuberculous endometritis, rare today in Western countries, is characterized by necrotizing granulomas containing acid-fast bacilli.

Microscopically, chronic endometritis should be suspected in biopsies that cannot be properly dated or seem to be out of date with the menstrual cycle or shows glandular- stromal asynchrony. The diagnosis is based on finding plasma cells in the stroma (Fig. 4.8). The salient features of chronic nonspecific endometritis are summarized in Box 4.3.

Hormonally Induced Changes

1. *Dysfunctional uterine bleeding (DUB):* It is a clinical term used for excessive menstrual or abnormal intermenstrual hemorrhage. It may be caused by *pathologic changes in the uterus,* but often it is related to *functional endocrine* changes or *systemic disease* without any specific anatomic basis.

Box 4.3. Chronic "nonspecific" endometritis

ETIOLOGY
- Usually no specific pathogens identified
- Associated with abortion, intrauterine device or pelvic inflammatory disease

CLINICAL FEATURES
- Vaginal bleeding
- Pelvic pain

PATHOLOGY
- Stromal infiltrates of plasma cells *
- Inflammatory cells in the glands
- Stellate endometrial stromal cells around glands in a pinwheel arrangement

---

*Pearl: The presence of lymphocytes or lymphoid follicles in the endometrial mucosa should not be considered as evidence of chronic endometritis

---

Anovulatory cycle is probably the most common cause of DUB. Most often it is encountered in prepubertal girls and premenopausal women. If the ovulation does not occur for whatever reasons around day 14 of the menstrual cycle, the unruptured follicles in the ovary continue to secrete estrogens, which continuously stimulate the proliferation of the endometrium. When the thickness of the endometrium exceeds the blood supply, the surface of the endometrial lining of the uterus becomes ischemic and bleeding occurs. Endometrial biopsy typically contains fragmented endometrial glands that are in a proliferative phase and are surrounded by condensed stromal cells in a background of hemorrhage and thrombosis. Focally there is crowding of glands.

Stellate stromal cells

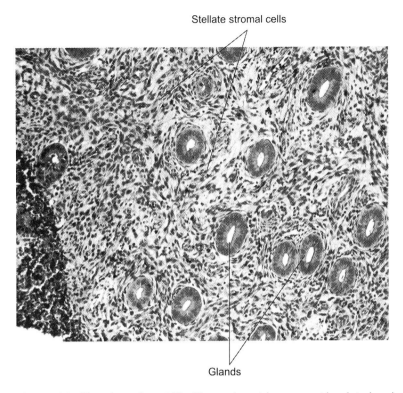

Glands

Figure 4.8. Chronic endometritis: The endometrium cannot be dated and consists of small glands surrounded by edematous stroma. Stellate stromal cells are typically seen. There are also scattered plasma cells, but these cannot be recognized at this low magnification.

These changes are also called "glandular and stromal breakdown." Surface epithelium may show cells that have indistinct borders typical of so-called syncytial metaplasia is often present on the surface.

Inadequate luteal phase due to poorly developed corpus luteum or early regression also may cause uterine bleeding. The endometrium may show a discordance in the maturation of glands and stroma (Fig. 4.9). However, the microscopic changes are often quite variable.

2. *Endometrial atrophy:* It accounts for 80 percent of postmenopausal bleeding. The endometrium is thin containing small glands that are often cystically dilated and surrounded by scant compact stroma (Fig. 4.10). The glands are lined by a single layer of flattened or cuboidal cells without mitosis. The biopsy specimen often contains very little tissue.

Exogenous administration of hormones may induce recognizable microscopic changes as follows:

• *Estrogen*: It will induce proliferation of endometrium and may cause endometrial hyperplasia. Prolonged administration is associated with increased risk of endometrial adenocarcinoma.

• *Tamoxifen:* It has a paradoxical estrogenic effect on endometrium, especially in postmenopausal women. It is associated with endometrial hyperplasia, polyps, and occasionally even carcinoma. Tamoxifen induced polyps contain branching " staghorn-shaped" glands and glands lined in parallel with the long axis of the polyps. Stromal condensation alternates with stroma condensation leading to the formation of a superficial subepithelial " cambium layer." Epithelial metaplasia and stromal myxoid degeneration are common (Fig. 4.11).

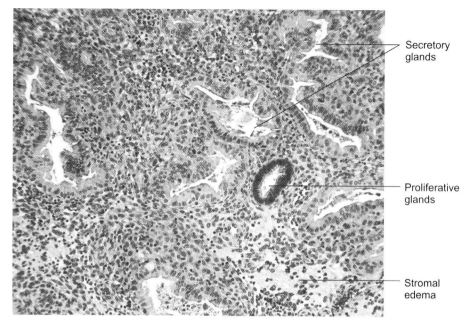

Figure 4.9. Dysfunctional uterine bleeding due to insufficient luteal phase. Some glands are in secretory phase and other in proliferative phase. The stroma is proliferative.

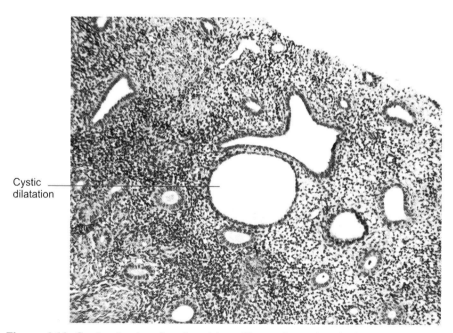

Figure 4.10. Cystic atrophy of endometrium: The endometrium is thin and contains cystically dilated glands surrounded by diminished endometrial stroma. Endometrium atrophy is the most common cause of postmenopausal bleeding.

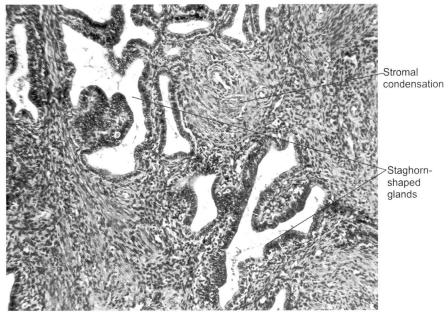

Figure 4.11. Tamoxifen effect: Staghorn-shaped glands with variable periglandular stromal condensation are typically found.

Stromal condensation

Staghorn-shaped glands

- *Progesterone:* Typically it affects both the stroma and the glands, but the effect depends on the agents and regimen used. In general, progesterone induces marked pseudodecidualization of the endometrial stroma and the glands are small and inactive (Fig. 4.12).
3. *Endometrial hyperplasia:* It refers to proliferation of glands with an increased gland to stroma ratio as compared to the proliferative endometrium. Although most likely caused by hormones, the real cause and pathogenesis of these changes are not always known. In many cases endometrial hyperplasia may progress to neoplasia. Clinically, endometrial hyperplasia typically present with abnormal bleeding.

The classification by the World Health Organization (WHO) takes into account both the cytologic and the architectural abnormalities. Two broad categories of endometrial hyperplasia are recognized: endometrial hyperplasia without atypia and endometrial hyperplasia with atypia. On the basis of their architectural complexity these two forms of endometrial hyperplasia are subclassified as simple or complex (Box 4.4). The rationale behind this classification is that hyperplasia with cytologic atypia has a higher risk to progress to carcinoma as compared to hyperplasia without atypia. The degree of architectural complexity adds to the likelihood of progression to neoplasia.

- *Simple hyperplasia without atypia*: It is characterized by abundant tubular endometrial glands which show occasional outpouching and focal crowding. The glandular cells are columnar, pseudostratified with variable mitosis lacking atypia (Fig. 4.13).
- *Complex hyperplasia without atypia*: It is characterized by branching glands showing irregular epithelial budding and papillary infolding. Glands compressing the surrounding

Box 4.4. Classification of endometrial hyperplasia

HYPERPLASIA (TYPICAL)
- Simple hyperplasia without atypia
- Complex hyperplasia without atypia

ATYPICAL HYPERPLASIA
- Simple atypical hyperplasia
- Complex atypical hyperplasia

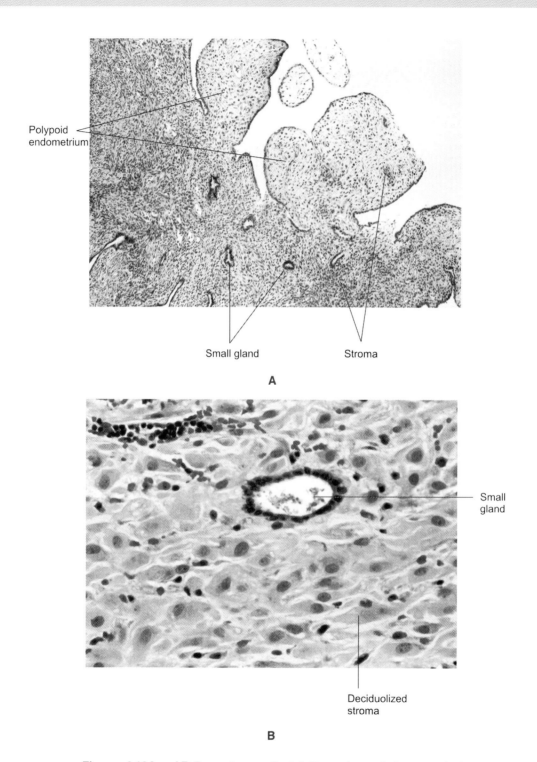

Polypoid endometrium

Small gland

Stroma

A

Small gland

Deciduolized stroma

B

Figures 4.12A and B. Progesterone effect: A. Progesterone induces marked pseudodecidualization of the endometrial stroma, sometimes forming a polypoid appearance. The glands are small and inactive. B. High power shows decidualized stromal cells with abundant eosinophilic cytoplasm and indistinct cell borders.

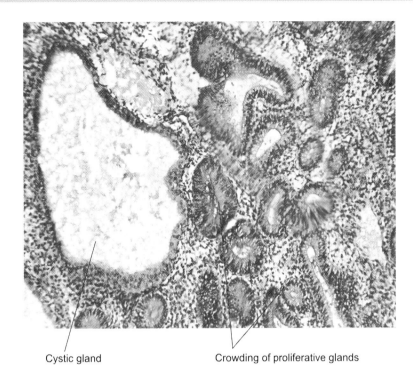

Cystic gland   Crowding of proliferative glands

Figure 4.13. Endometrial simple hyperplasia without atypia. The glands are cystically dilated with no significant outpouching or infolding. There is no cytologic atypia in the glandular lining epithelial cells.

stroma appear crowded and are arranged "back-to-back". There is no or only minimal cellular atypia (Fig. 4.14).

- *Atypical hyperplasia*: It has many features of simple or complex hyperplasia but also shows prominent nuclear atypia. The nuclei lose their normal polarity. They have prominent nucleoli, and show chromatin clearing. The nuclear outlines are irregular (Fig. 4.15). Atypical hyperplasia may gradually progress to endometrial carcinoma, from which it cannot be always distinguished with certainty.

Neoplasms

Endometrial carcinoma is the most common malignancy of female gynecologic tract in developed countries. Most carcinomas (80%) occur in postmenopausal women (Box 4.5).

On gross examination the tumors are exophytic protruding into the uterine cavity and invasive, penetrating into the myometrium (Fig. 4.16). Some tumors present as diffuse endometrial thickening, whereas others form solitary polypoid masses or ulcerations (Box 4.6).

Endometrial polyp is a benign lesion that protrudes into the endometrial cavity (Fig. 4.17). Histologically, it is composed of endometrial glands and stroma. The glandular component is usually patchily distributed with some cystic changes. The stroma is fibrous and characteristically contains thick-walled, tortuous, dilated blood vessels (Fig. 4.18). Most endometrial polyps are benign, but some may contain foci of endometrial carcinoma.

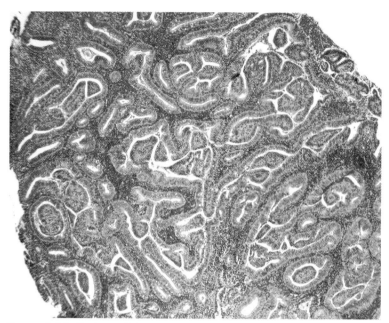

Figure 4.14. Endometrial complex hyperplasia without atypia. There is marked gland crowding with minimal intervening stroma (back-to-back glands). Cytologic atypia is absent.

Box 4.5. Endometrial carcinoma

ETIOLOGY
- Estrogen effect
- Genetic alterations
  - *PTEN, TP 53 or K-ras* mutation
- Microsatellite instability

CLASSIFICATION
- Type I -related to estrogen
- Type II- unrelated to estrogen

CLINICAL FEATURES
- Peak incidence in the 55-65 years age group
- Spotting
- Menorrhagia
- Metrorrhagia
- Postmenopausal bleeding

TREATMENT
- Surgery

Box 4.6. Macroscopic pathology of endometrial adenocarcinoma

- Enlarged uterus
- Diffuse thickening of endometrium*
- Exophytic, polypoid mass
- Ulcerated endometrial surface

Pearl: Thickening of the endometrium may be recognized by ultrasound

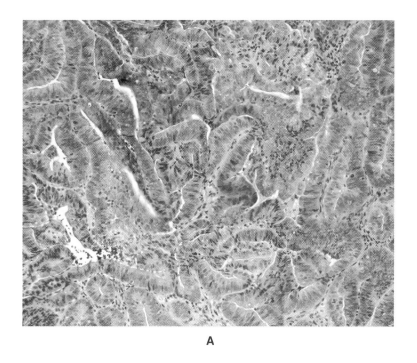

A

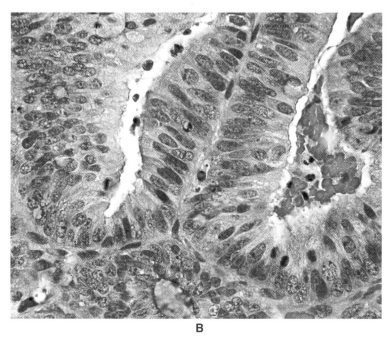

B

Figures 4.15A and B. Endometrial complex hyperplasia with atypia: A. There is marked back-to-back appearance with glandular branching and infolding. The cells are hyperchromatic with loss of polarity. B. High power shows the cytologic atypia including loss of polarity, hyperchromatic nuclei with irregular nuclear membrane, prominent nucleoli and frequent mitosis.

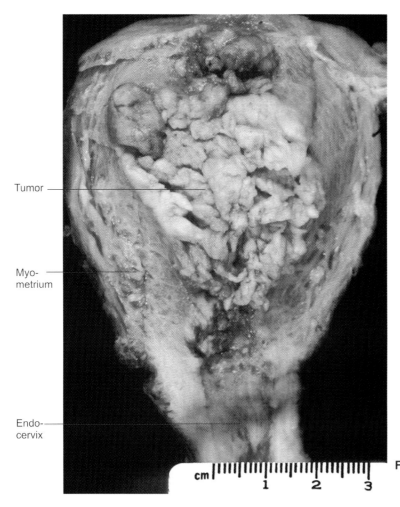

Tumor

Myo-
metrium

Endo-
cervix

cm | 1 2 3

Figure 4.16. Endometrial adenocarcinoma: The exophytic tumor fills the endometrial cavity.

Based on pathogenesis, endometrial carcinoma can be divided into two categories: those associated with high estrogenic status (type I) and those that are independent of estrogen status of the patient (type II). Risk factors for the first category include obesity, diabetes, nulliparity, hypertension and late menopause. The estrogen-dependent tumors are usually low-grade with minimal myometrial invasion. Histologically, they are usually of the endometrioid type and frequently associated with endometrial hyperplasia. Type II endometrial carcinomas are usually high-grade tumors showing deep myometrial invasion and aggressive clinical behavior. Histologic forms of endometrial adenocarcinoma are listed in Box 4.7.

1. *Endometrioid adenocarcinoma:* It is the most common type of endometrial carcinoma. It is composed of neoplastic glands resembling those of the normal endometrium (Fig. 4.19). The distinction between well-differentiated endometrioid adenocarcinoma and atypical complex hyperplasia may be difficult and at times impossible. In such cases one must look for subtle clues favoring malignancy such as a stromal desmoplastic response, tumor necrosis and confluent cribriform patterns of glands.

   Endometrioid carcinoma may present in several variant forms which, however, have the same prognosis as the typical endometrioid carcinoma. The most important variants of endometrioid carcinoma are listed as follows:

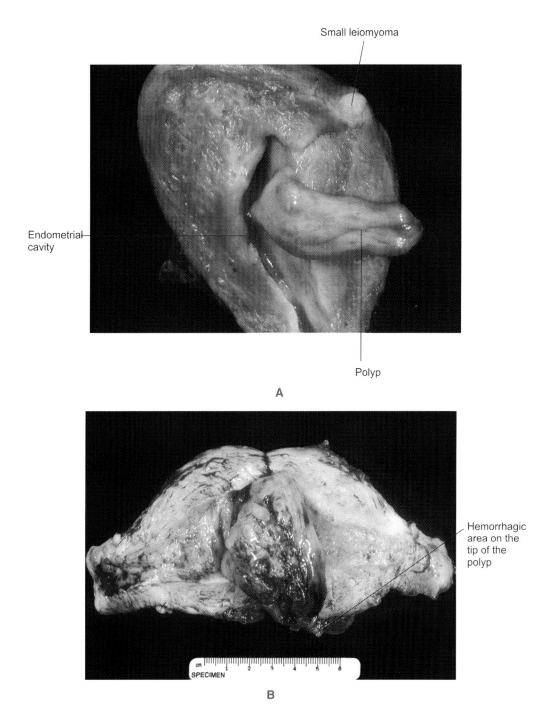

Small leiomyoma

Endometrial cavity

Polyp

A

Hemorrhagic area on the tip of the polyp

B

Figures 4.17A and B. Endometrial polyp: A. Endometrial polyp protrudes into the endometrial cavity. B. Area of hemorrhage and necrosis maybe present on the surface of endometrial polyp.

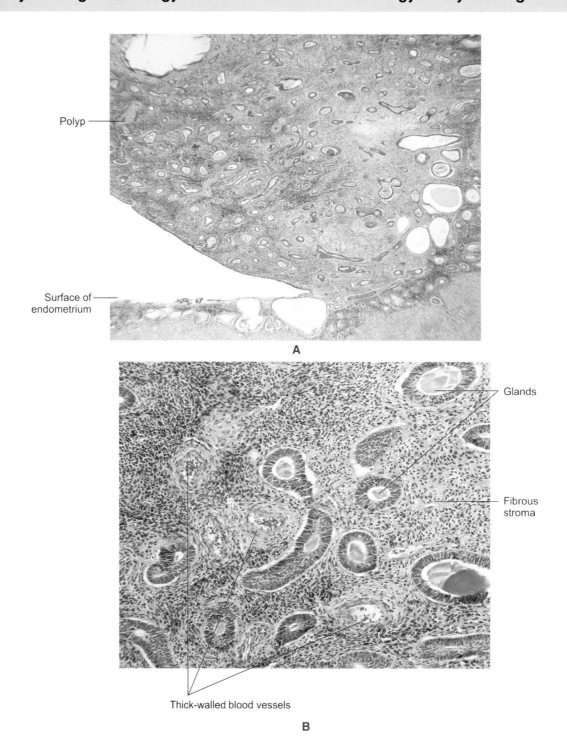

Polyp

Surface of endometrium

A

Glands

Fibrous stroma

Thick-walled blood vessels

B

Figures 4.18A and B. Endometrial polyp: A. Low-power view shows the polypoid lesion containing both endometrial glands and stroma protruding above the surface of endometrial cavity. B. The stroma is usually fibrous and contains thick-walled blood vessels.

Box 4.7. Microscopic types of endometrial adenocarcinoma

- Endometrioid adenocarcinoma
  - Variant with squamous differentiation
  - Villoglandular variant
  - Secretory variant
  - Ciliated cell variant
- Mucinous adenocarcinoma
- Serous adenocarcinoma
- Clear cell adenocarcinoma
- Squamous cell carcinoma
- Transitional cell carcinoma
- Small cell carcinoma
- Undifferentiated carcinoma

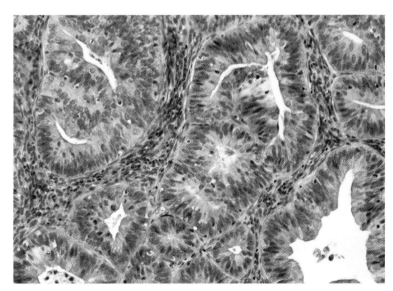

Figure 4.19. Endometrioid adenocarcinoma: This most common type of endometrial adenocarcinoma is composed of malignant glands resembling normal endometrial glands, but with complex architectural pattern, and marked cytologic atypia.

- *Endometrioid adenocarcinoma with squamous differentiation*: This tumor is composed of typical endometrioid carcinoma with scattered foci of squamous metaplasia or carcinoma (Fig. 4.20A). The squamous or morular component should not be considered as a solid part of the tumor when evaluating the architectural grade.
- *Villoglandular variant of endometrioid carcinoma*: It is characterized by thin and delicate papillary fronds and villi covered by columnar epithelium. The cells have nuclei of low or intermediate nuclear grade (Fig. 4.20B). This variant must be distinguished from the papillary serous carcinoma, a more malignant tumor that shows complex papillary architecture and is composed of cells that have a high nuclear grade.

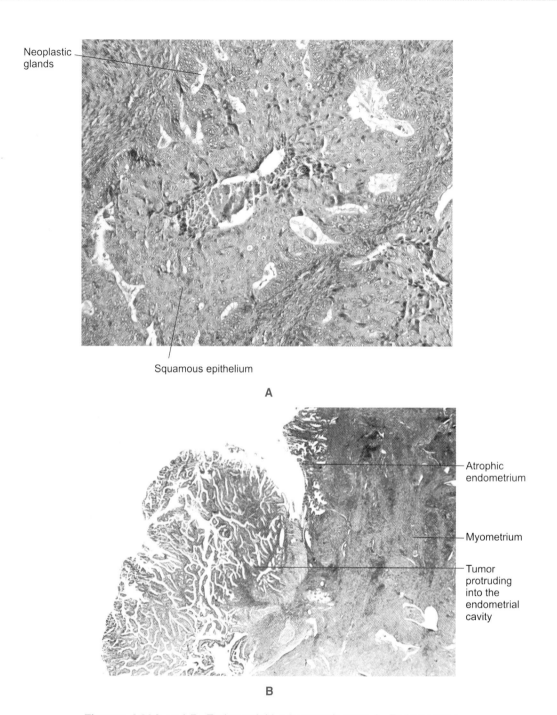

Neoplastic glands

Squamous epithelium

A

Atrophic endometrium

Myometrium

Tumor protruding into the endometrial cavity

B

Figures 4.20A and B. Endometrioid adenocarcinoma: A. Endometrioid carcinoma with squamous differentiation consists of glands and foci of squamous differentiation. B. Villoglandular variant of endometrioid carcinoma is characterized by an exophytic growth of thin and delicate papillary villi.

- *Secretory variant of endometrioid carcinomas*: It is composed of crowded glands that have a complex structure resembling secretory endometrium. Tumor cells have well developed clear cytoplasm and contain characteristic subnuclear glycogen vacuoles. The nuclei are low grade and appear bland.
- *Ciliated cell variant*: It is a rare form of low-grade endometrioid carcinoma containing ciliated cells resembling fallopian tube epithelium.

2. *Mucinous adenocarcinoma*: It is an uncommon type of endometrial carcinoma in which at least half of the tumor is composed of epithelial cells containing prominent intracytoplasmic mucin (Fig. 4.21). They are generally low-grade tumors with prognosis comparable to that of grade I endometrioid carcinomas.

3. *Serous adenocarcinoma*: It typifies the non-estrogen dependent (type II) endometrial carcinomas. Grossly, the tumor is usually exophytic, markedly papillary and friable. The histology of serous carcinoma is characterized by papillary structures with broad fibrovascular cores covered by highly malignant cells resembling ovarian papillary serous carcinoma (Fig. 4.22). Mitoses, solid cell nests, foci of necrosis and psammoma bodies are commonly present. Serous carcinoma is, by definition, a high-grade endometrial carcinoma associated with deep myometrial invasion, extensive angiolymphatic invasion, and extrauterine spread.

4. *Clear cell adenocarcinoma*: It is composed of large, clear, glycogen-filled and hobnail cells protruding into glandular lumens and papillary spaces (Fig. 4.23). Unlike the secretory variant of endometrioid carcinoma, the nuclei of clear cell carcinoma are highly pleomorphic with bizarre and multinucleated forms. Most patients with clear cell carcinoma are postmenopausal and are frequently diagnosed in advanced clinical stages. Unlike clear cell carcinoma of the vagina and cervix, there seems to be no relationship between endometrial clear cell carcinoma and intrauterine diethylstilbestrol exposure.

5. *Rare forms of carcinoma*: These forms deserve to be mentioned because these tumors may pose diagnostic problems and may be mistakenly diagnosed as metastases. This group includes the following tumor types:
   - *Squamous cell carcinoma*: This rare form of endometrial carcinoma resembles cervical cancer from which it must be distinguished.
   - *Transitional cell carcinoma*: This diagnosis is made when the endometrial carcinoma in which 90% or more of the tumor is composed of cells resembling urothelial epithelium. The tumor usually has a papillary configuration. The diagnosis should be made only after one has excluded the possibility of metastasis from the bladder or the ovary.
   - *Mixed adenocarcinoma*: This term is used for endometrial carcinomas with two or more epithelial components. The diagnosis of mixed adenocarcinoma is made only if the minor component accounts for at least 10% of the total volume of the tumor.

Prognosis of endometrial carcinoma depends on the tumor stage, depth of myometrial invasion, and the presence or absence of lymphovascular invasion, histologic type, histologic grade. Histologically, endometrial adenocarcinomas are graded using both nuclear and architectural criteria ("nuclear grade and architectural grade"), summarized in Boxes 4.8 and 4.9 and illustrated in Figures 4.24 and 4.25.

Mesenchymal Tumors

1. *Leiomyoma*: Clinically also known as "fibroid". It is a benign tumor composed of smooth muscle cells. It is the most common uterine tumor. Leiomyomas are more common in black women than in other races and tend to be multiple. On gross examination they appear well-circumscribed, rubbery, white nodular mass with whirled

Box 4.8. Nuclear grading of endometrial adenocarcinoma according to FIGO	Box 4.9. Architectural grading of endometrial adenocarcinoma according to FIGO
• Grade 1: Mildly enlarged, oval nuclei with evenly dispersed chromatin and no nucleoli. • Grade 2: Moderately enlarged nuclei with small nucleoli and variable mitotic activity. • Grade 3: Markedly enlarged and pleomorphic nuclei with irregular coarse chromatin, prominent nucleoli and frequent mitosis with atypical forms	• Grade 1 : No more than 5% (< 5%) of the tumor is composed of non-squamous, non-morular solid growth pattern. • Grade 2 : 6-50% of the tumor is composed of non-squamous, non-morular solid growth pattern. • Grade 3 : More than 50% of the tumor is composed of non-squamous, non-morular solid growth pattern.

Note: Bizarre nuclei should raise the architectural grade by one.

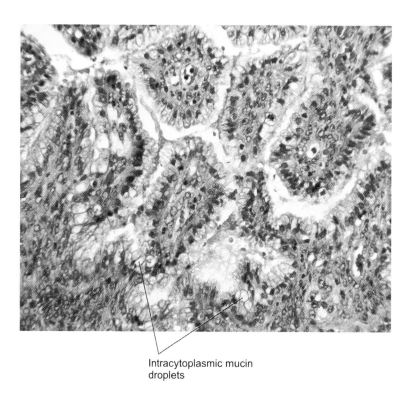

Intracytoplasmic mucin droplets

Figure 4.21. Mucinous adenocarcinoma: More than half of the tumor is composed of malignant epithelial cells containing intracytoplasmic mucin.

cut surface (Fig. 4.26). Cystic degeneration, hyalinization, calcification and hemorrhage may be seen. Microscopically, the tumors are composed of fascicles of uniform spindle cells with elongated, blunt-ended nuclei, fine chromatin, small nucleoli, and eosinophilic abundant cytoplasm (Fig. 4.27). Mitoses are infrequent (usually less than 5 per 10 high power fields). Hemorrhage, edema, myxoid degeneration, and hyaline fibrosis are common.

The clinical symptoms depend on the location which may be submucosal, intramural or subserosal (Boxes 4.10 and 4.11).

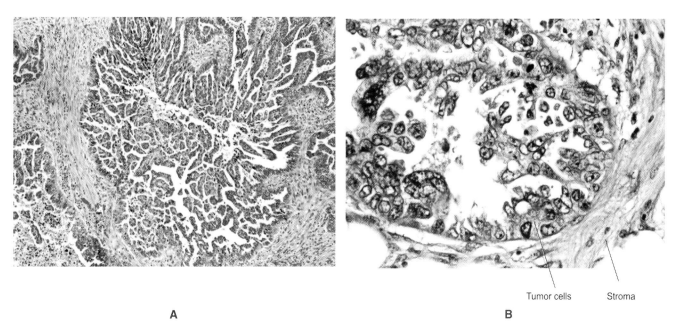

A

B

Tumor cells   Stroma

Figures 4.22A and B. Serous adenocarcinoma: A. This high-grade endometrial carcinoma usually has a papillary configuration with broad fibrovascular cores covered by highly malignant cells. B. The cells are highly pleomorphic with frequent mitosis and atypical forms. Tumor necrosis and psammoma bodies are usually seen.

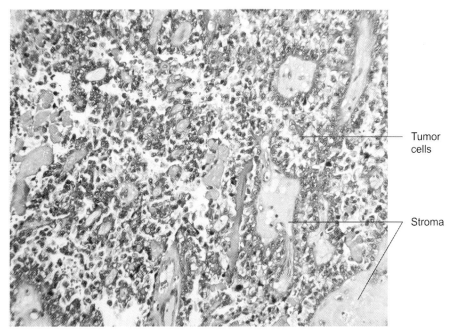

Tumor cells

Stroma

Figure 4.23. Clear cell adenocarcinoma: This tumor is composed of large, clear and hobnail cells protruding into glandular lumens. The cells are markedly pleomorphic and there are frequent mitoses.

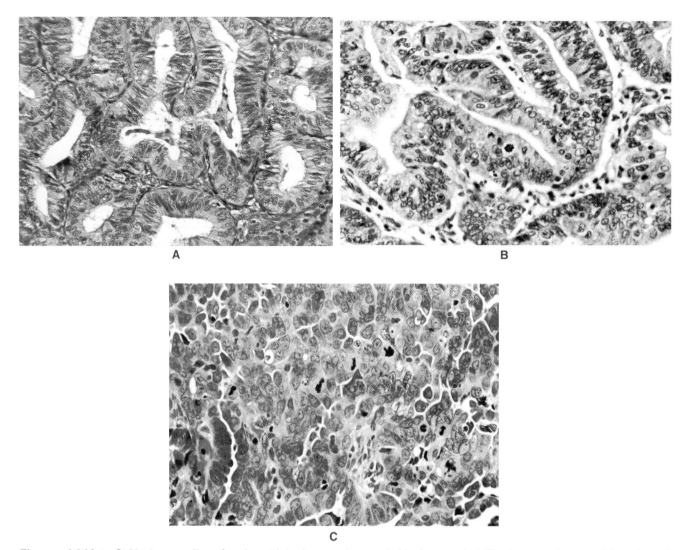

Figures 4.24A to C. Nuclear grading of endometrial adenocarcinoma: A. Nuclear grade I. The tumor cells are mildly enlarged with oval nuclei and have no nucleoli. B. Nuclear grade II. The tumor cell nuclei are moderately enlarged and contain small nucleoli. There are mitoses in variable numbers. C. Nuclear grade III. The tumor cells nuclei are markedly enlarged. They have pleomorphic nuclei and coarse chromatin, prominent nucleoli. There are numerous mitoses.

Box 4.10. Clinical features of uterine leiomyomas	Box 4.11. Macroscopic pathology of uterine leiomyomas
EPIDEMIOLOGY	LOCATION
• Tumor of reproductive age	• Submucosal
• More common in black women than other races	• Intramural
CLINICAL FEATURES	• Subserosal
• Asymptomatic	SIZE AND SHAPE
• Bleeding, metrorrhagia, menorrhagia	• Size varies from 1 to 30 cm
• Pain and discomfort	• Consistency firm and rubbery
• Compression of other pelvic organs	• Cross section appears whorled
	• May be edematous, soft, cystic
	• Postmenopausal tumors tend to shrink
	• Secondary hyalinization and calcification

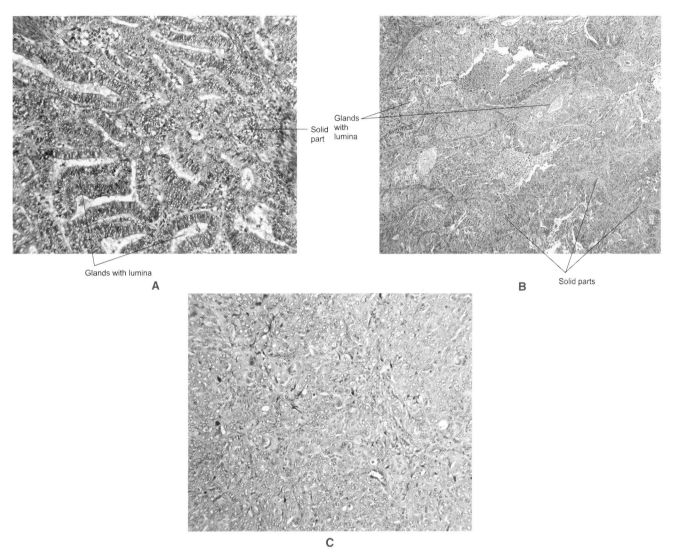

Figures 4.25A to C. Architectural grading of endometrial adenocarcinoma: A. Architectural grade I—Less than 5% of the tumor is composed of solid growth pattern. B. Architectural grade II—6-50% of the tumor shows solid growth. C. Architectural grade III—More than 50% of the tumor shows solid growth.

Variant forms of leiomyoma that are clinically important include the following entities:

- *Cellular leiomyoma*: This variant of leiomyoma characterized by markedly increased cellularity compared to the surrounding myometrium (Fig. 4.28). Lack of tumor necrosis, lack of significant atypia and infrequent mitotic figures in the cellular leiomyoma differentiate it from leiomyosarcoma.
- *Mitotically active leiomyoma*: This tumor has all the typical features of leiomyoma but shows increased mitotic activity (> 5 per 10 high power fields). This diagnosis should be limited to tumors with no marked nuclear atypia, no atypical mitosis, and no tumor necrosis.

2. *Smooth muscle tumor of uncertain malignant potential (STUMP)*: It is a category comprising tumors that cannot be diagnosed with certainty as benign or malignant because of ambiguous histology features. In general, tumors are regarded as leiomyosarcoma when they have coagulative necrosis, high mitotic activity (greater

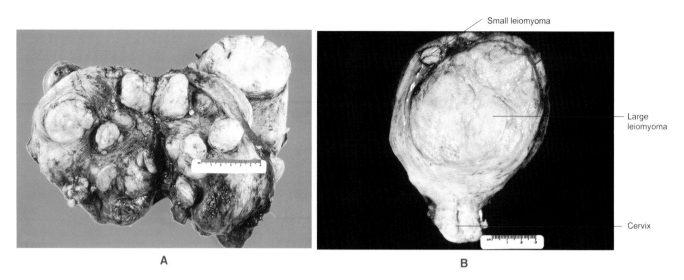

Figures 4.26A and B. Leiomyoma: A. The myometrium contains several well-circumscribed, rubbery, white nodular masses. B. The cut surface of this large leiomyoma has a whorled appearance. A small satellite leiomyoma is seen the myometrium as well.

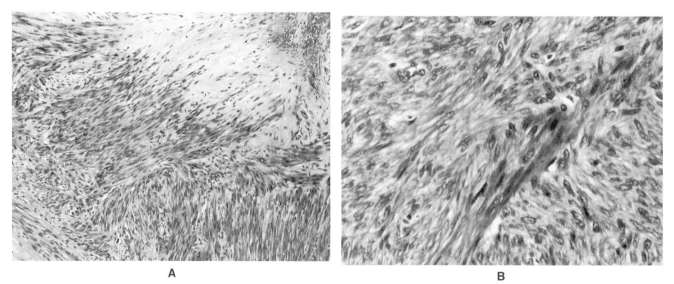

Figures 4.27A and B. Leiomyoma: A. Fascicles of uniform spindle cells with eosinophilic cytoplasm are typical of smooth muscle cells. B. Tumor cells have elongated, blunt-ended nuclei, uniformly dispersed chromatin, inconspicuous nucleoli, and abundant eosinophilic cytoplasm.

than 10 per 10 HPF) and diffuse atypia. When a tumor contains foci of coagulative necrosis, but lacks diffuse atypia and increased mitotic activity, or has increased mitotic activity and focal atypia but lacks diffuse atypia and necrosis, or has diffuse atypia, but lack coagulative necrosis and increased mitotic activity, it is placed under this category.

3. *Leiomyosarcoma:* It is the most common uterine sarcoma. It almost exclusively occurs in adults. Clinically it may present as a rapidly growing uterus after menopause, or abdominal mass and gastrointestinal or urinary

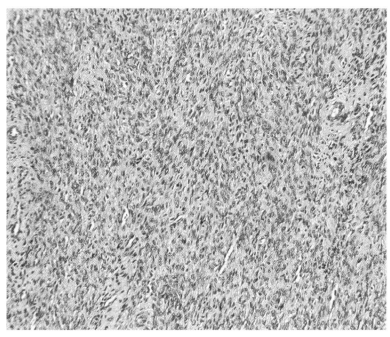

Figure 4.28. Cellular leiomyoma: The tumor is hypercellular but shows no mitotic activity and contains no foci of necrosis.

tract symptoms. Grossly, the tumor is large (average 8.0 cm) with poorly defined margins. The tumor cut surface is fleshy with areas of hemorrhage and necrosis (Fig. 4.29). Microscopically, leiomyosarcoma is hypercellular and composed pleomorphic hyperchromic cells (Fig. 4.30). There are usually more than 15 mitoses per 10 high power fields. Coagulative tumor necrosis is typically present. Vascular invasion is identified in up to one-fourth of the cases.

4. *Endometrial stromal tumors (ESS):* They are composed of small blue cells resembling normal proliferating endometrial stroma. These tumors are usually diagnosed in middle-aged women. Based on the tumor margins (pushing verus infiltrating) and presence or absence of vascular invasion, ESS are divided into two groups : benign endometrial stromal nodules and endometrial stromal sarcoma. Endometrial stromal sarcoma is further subdivided into two groups: low-grade tumors and undifferentiated high grade tumors.

a. **Endometrial stromal nodules:** They are grossly well-circumscribed intramural nodular masses with soft, tan to yellow cut surfaces. Histology shows small bland ovoid cells with indistinct cytoplasm (Fig. 4.31) and strong immunoreactivity with antibodies to CD10. No myometrial invasion or angiolymphatic invasion is present. The prognosis is good.

b. **Low-grade endometrial stromal sarcoma:** It is distinguished from the endometrial stromal nodules by the presence of myometrial and lymphovascular invasions. The low-power view is distinctive showing extensive permeation of myometrium by tumor islands. The tumor is highly cellular with packed ovoid to spindle tumor cells (Fig. 4.32). Pleomorphism and mitosis are variable. Low-grade endometrial stromal sarcoma has an indolent growth and may develop local recurrence and distant metastases to the lung.

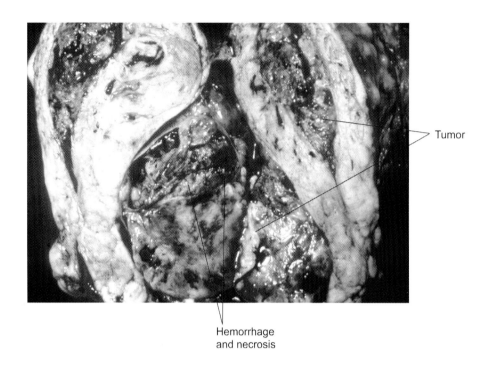

Tumor

Hemorrhage
and necrosis

Figure 4.29. Leiomyosarcoma: The bulky tumor fills the uterine cavity. On cross-section it contains prominent areas of hemorrhage and necrosis.

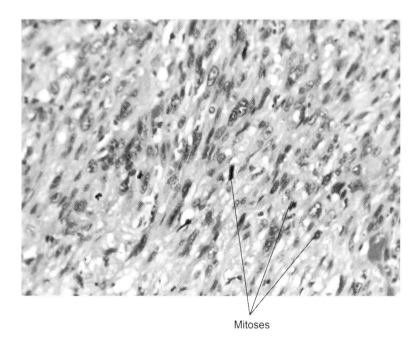

Mitoses

Figure 4.30. Leiomyosarcoma: The tumor is hypercellular, shows brisk mitotic activity and contains foci of necrosis.

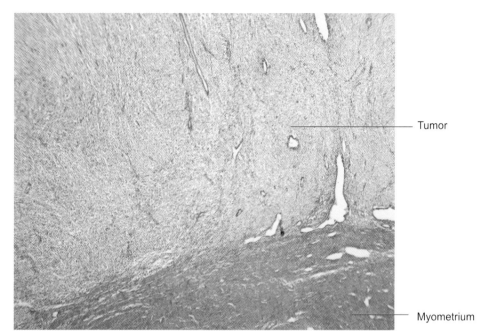

Tumor

Myometrium

Figure 4.31. Endometrial stromal nodule: The tumor is composed of small bland endometrial stromal cells forming a well-circumscribed intramural nodule. No myometrial or lymphovascular invasion is present.

c. **Undifferentiated endometrial sarcoma:** It shows histologically signs of anaplasia such as marked cellular pleomorphism, frequent mitosis and often atypical nuclei. There are prominent foci of tumor necrosis (Fig. 4.33). It lacks specific differentiation either morphologically or immunohistochemically. The prognosis is poor.

Mixed Epithelial and Mesenchymal Tumors

Mixed epithelial and mesenchymal tumors may benign or malignant. Benign tumors include adenomyomas and adenofibromas, whereas the malignant tumor group includes adenosarcomas and carcinosarcomas. Clinically, the most important tumor in this group is carcinosarcoma.

Carcinosarcoma, or *malignant mixed müllerian tumor (MMMT)* is a neoplasm composed of malignant epithelial and malignant mesenchymal components. It usually occurs in postmenopausal women and presents as vaginal bleeding. It may also present as polypoid necrotic mass protruding through the cervix.

On gross examination carcinosarcomas are usually exophytic and form bulky masses that fill the uterine cavity and invade deeply into myometrium (Fig. 4.34). Areas of necrosis and hemorrhage are common. The malignant epithelial component has the microscopic features of adenocarcinoma, which may be of endometrioid, serous or clear cell type (Fig. 4.35A). The sarcomatous component may be homologous or heterologous. The homologous stroma is composed of cells that are normally present in the uterus and accordingly it may have the microscopic features of endometrial stromal sarcoma, leiomyosarcoma, or undifferentiated sarcoma (Fig. 4.35B). The

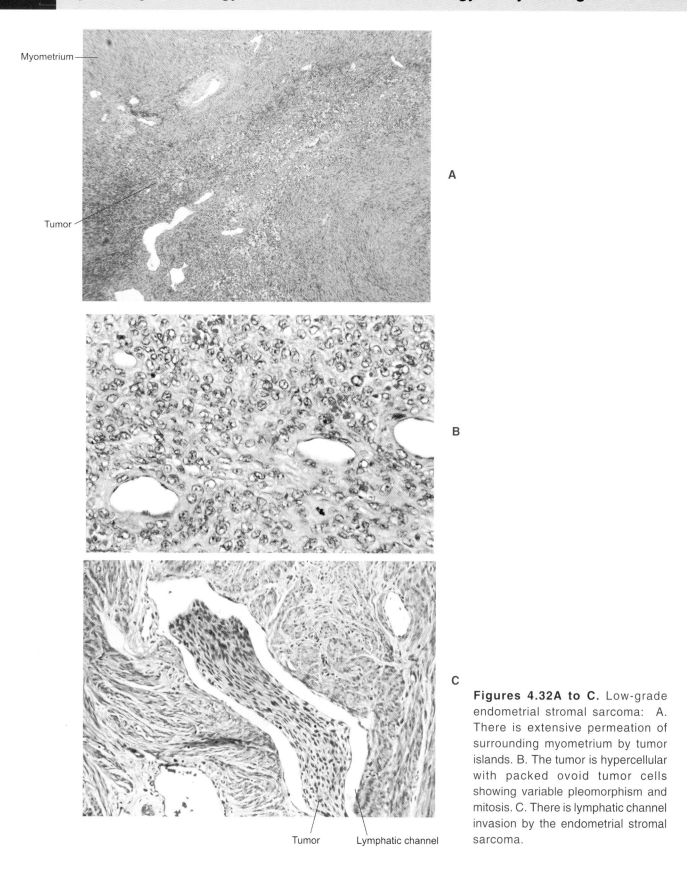

Myometrium

Tumor

A

B

C

Tumor   Lymphatic channel

Figures 4.32A to C. Low-grade endometrial stromal sarcoma: A. There is extensive permeation of surrounding myometrium by tumor islands. B. The tumor is hypercellular with packed ovoid tumor cells showing variable pleomorphism and mitosis. C. There is lymphatic channel invasion by the endometrial stromal sarcoma.

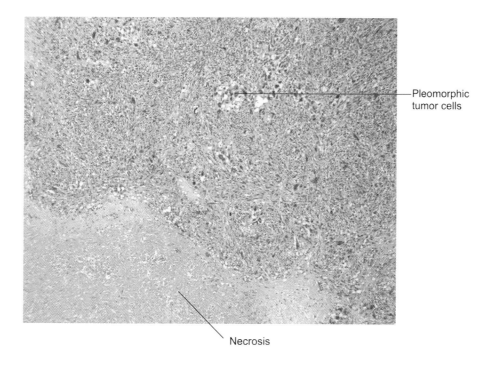

Pleomorphic
tumor cells

Necrosis

Figure 4.33. Undifferentiated endometrial sarcoma. The tumor has marked pleomorphism, frequent mitosis with atypical forms and extensive tumor necrosis. It generally lacks specific differentiation morphologically or immunohistochemically.

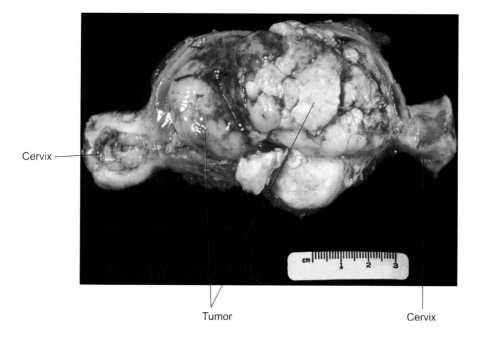

Cervix

Tumor   Cervix

Figure 4.34. Carcinosarcoma: The tumor consists of bulky exophytic masses showing foci of necrosis and also invading into the myometrium.

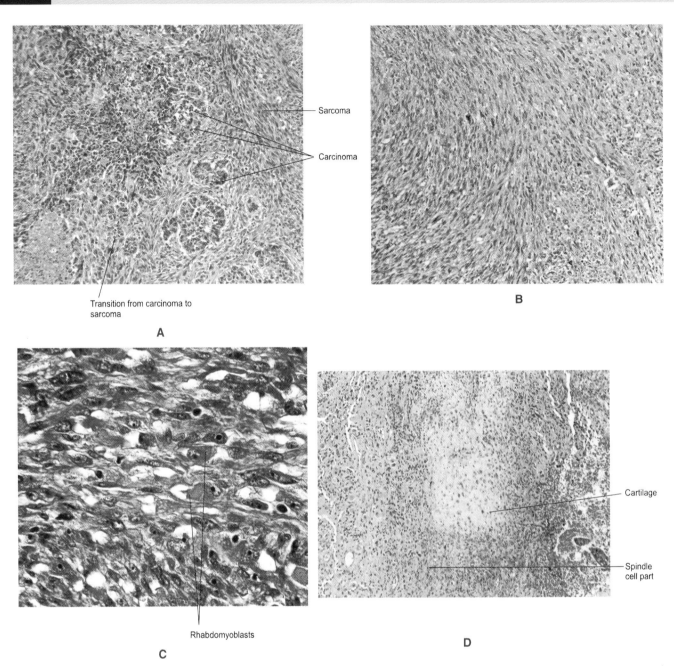

Sarcoma

Carcinoma

Transition from carcinoma to
sarcoma

A

B

Rhabdomyoblasts

C

Cartilage

Spindle
cell part

D

Figures 4.35A to D. Carcinosarcoma: A. The tumor consists of epithelial (carcinomatous) and mesenchymal (sarcomatous) components. B. This homologous stromal component has the microscopic features of leiomyosarcoma. C. This heterologous component contains immature skeletal muscle cells (rhabdomyoblasts) and has the microscopic features of rhabdomyosarcoma. D. This heterologous stromal component contains neoplastic cartilage and has the features of chondrosarcoma.

heterologous stroma consists of cell type that are not normally found in the uterus and accordingly it may have the microscopic features of chondrosarcoma, rhabdomyosarcoma, or less often osteosarcoma and liposarcoma (Figs 4.35C and D). Areas of transition between the epithelial and mesenchymal components may be identified. Carcinosarcomas are clinically aggressive tumors with poor prognosis.

5

Fallopian Tube

NORMAL ANATOMY AND HISTOLOGY

The fallopian tube is a hollow tubular structure that is located between the uterine cornus and the ovary (Fig. 5.1). It measures 11 to 12 cm in length and is embedded in the upper part of the broad ligament.

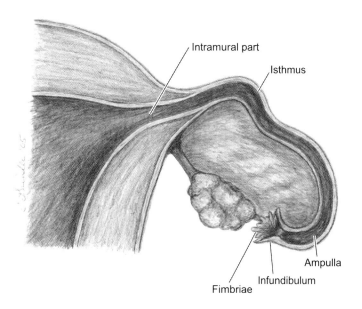

Figure 5.1. Normal fallopian tube has four parts known as the intramural, isthmic, infundibular, and ampullar portions.

The fallopian tube may be divided into four parts known as *the intramural part, isthmus, ampulla,* and *infundibulum.* The intramural part lies inside the uterine wall. The isthmus is a thick-walled and narrow portion, whereas the ampulla is a thin-walled expanded part of the tube. The infundibulum is the lateral end-part that opens into the peritoneal cavity through the ostium. It is fringed by fimbriae, which attach it loosely to the ovary.

Histologically, the fallopian tube wall consists of three layers: mucosa, muscularis and serosa. The *mucosa* is arranged into longitudinal branching folds known as plicae. It contains three types of cells: secretory, ciliated and intercalated cells (Fig. 5.2). The *muscularis* is composed of an inner circular layer and an outer longitudinal layer. The *serosa* is lined by flattened mesothelial cells.

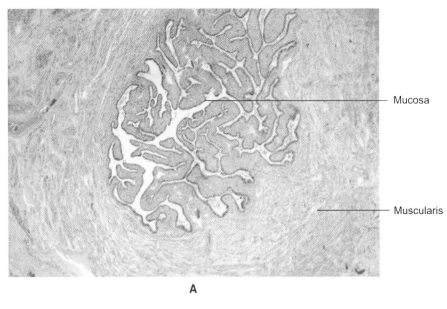

A

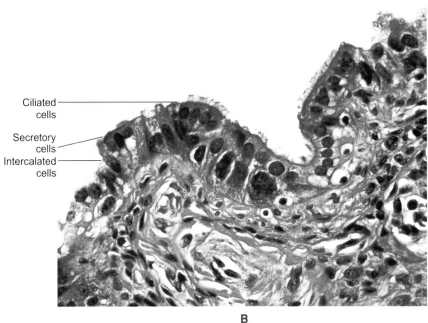

B

Figures 5.2A and B. Histology of normal fallopian tube: A. The fallopian tube wall is composed of mucosa, muscularis and serosa. The mucosa is arranged into branching folds known as plicae. B. High power view shows three types of cells lining the mucosa: secretory, ciliated and intercalated cells.

The fallopian tube plays an important role in the fertilization process. The synchronized motion of cilia and contractions of muscle layers help to pick up the ovulated ovum, the epithelial cells and secretions provide perfect microenvironment for retaining spermatozoa, the ovum and finally the fertilization, and eventually move the fertilized ovum to the uterus for implantation.

OVERVIEW OF PATHOLOGY

The most important diseases of the fallopian tubes are classified as follows:
• Non-neoplastic lesions
• Neoplasms

Non-neoplastic Lesions

1. *Salpingitis:* Also known as inflammation of the fallopian tubes, it can be acute or chronic. It is in most instances caused by polymicrobial infection. Such an infection is often superimposed on an initial sexually transmitted infection with *Neisseria gonorrhoeae* or *Chlamydia trachomatis*. On gross examination the infected tubes are swollen and red. Chronic inflammation is associated with fibrous adhesion with adjacent organs and gross distortion of the fallopian tubes. Microscopically one may recognize three forms of inflammation:
   • *Suppurative inflammation*: In this inflammation the lumen contains pus and the plicae are edematous and infiltrated with neutrophils.
   • *Nonspecific chronic inflammation:* Plicae are broadened and blunted and infiltrated with macrophages, lymphocytes and plasma cells (Fig. 5.3).
   • *Granulomatous salpingitis*: This form of inflammation is usually caused by *Mycobacterium tuberculosis*. Plicae contain granulomas which are composed of epithelioid macrophages, lymphocytes and multinucleated giant cells. Granulomatous salpingitis can also be seen in Crohn's disease and sarcoidosis (Fig. 5.4).

   The complications of salpingitis result from the extension of the inflammation or abortive healing of the chronic inflammation. The most important complications include the following lesions:
   • *Tubo-ovarian abscess*: The extension of the suppurative inflammation into the adjacent structures results in the formation of an adnexal mass comprising numerous fibrotic pus filled cavities, convoluted fallopian tube, mesosalpinx and the ovary (Fig. 5.5).
   • *Peritonitis*: Transmural inflammation or the outflow of pus into the abdominal activity from the orifices on the fimbrial end the tubes lead, to inflammation of the peritoneum. It may be localized to the pelvis or diffuse.
   • *Hydrosalpinx:* Healing of salpingitis may lead to fibrous occlusion of the fallopian tube and accumulation of serous fluid in its lumen (Fig. 5.6).
2. *Torsion of the fallopian tube*: Twisting of the tubes usually results from pathologic enlargement of the ovaries cause by tumors or tubal adhesions resulting from salpingitis. Clinically it presents as a sudden onset of lower abdominal pain. The adnexa are often edematous and the entire fallopian tube may appear infarcted.
3. *Endometriosis:* Implants of endometrial mucosa may be found on the serosa of the fallopian tubes or in the muscle layer. They appear as small red dots or nodules. Microscopically, these foci consist of endometrial glands and stroma, which usually contain extravasated blood.

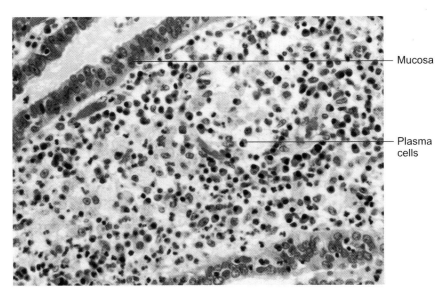

Figure 5.3. Chronic salpingitis: The plicae is broadened and blunted by macrophages, plasma cells and lymphocytes.

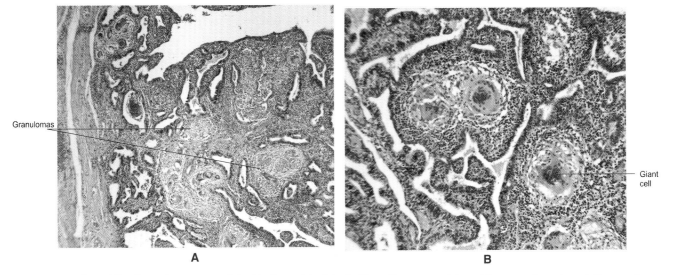

Figures 5.4A and B. Granulomatous salpingitis (sarcoidosis): A. The plicae are widened by granulomatous inflammation. B. Multinucleated giant cells are part of the granulomatous inflammation.

4. *Endosalpingiosis:* It is the presence of tubal-like epithelium in the peritoneum and serosal surfaces of the uterus and ovaries. In contrast to endometriosis, the glands are not surrounded by endometrial stroma and there is no stromal hemorrhage (Fig. 5.7).

5. *Tubal pregnancy:* It is the most common form of extrauterine pregnancy. The reasons for the intratubal implantation are not fully understood. It is nevertheless well known that tubal pregnancy occurs at in increased rate in women with congenital uterine or tubal anomalies, those who had preexisting chronic salpingitis, as well as those who have salpingitis isthmica nodosa. Clinically, tubal pregnancy presents with pelvic pain .The rupture of the tube may cause intraperitoneal bleeding and hypotensive shock. Following implantation of the ovum in

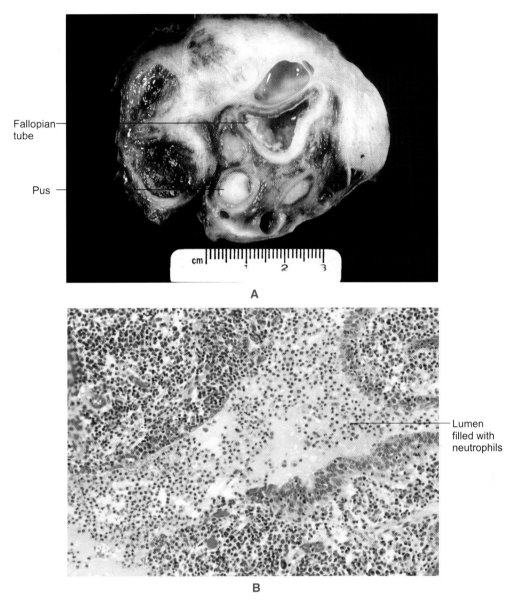

Figures 5.5A and B. Tubo-ovarian abscess: A. On cross section of the abscess one may see several cavities corresponding to the lumen of the convoluted fallopian tube and peritubal abscesses. Fibrous tissue forms broad strands obliterating the normal outlines of the ovary and the fallopian tubes. B. Microscopically, the wall and the lumen of the fallopian tube contains neutrophils.

the tube (usually in the ampullar-isthmic portion), chorionic villi and intermediate trophoblasts may grow predominantly within the lumen or penetrate deeply into the wall of the fallopian tube. On gross examination the fallopian tube appears dilated and is filled with blood (hematosalpinx). The fetus or placental chorionic villi can be often identified (Fig. 5.8). Microscopically, chorionic villi are seen penetrating into the muscular wall (Fig. 5.9).

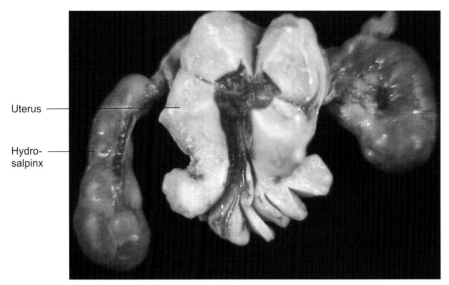

Uterus

Hydro-
salpinx

Figure 5.6. Hydrosalpinx: A. Both fallopian tubes are dilated and filled with fluid.

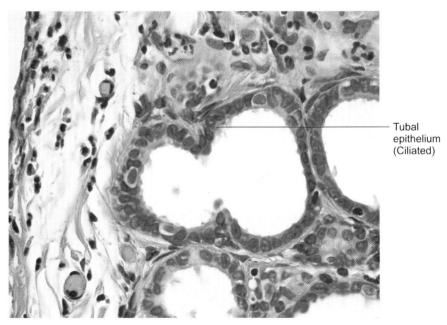

Tubal
epithelium
(Ciliated)

Figure 5.7. Endosalpingiosis: The glands are lined by epithelium resembling normal tubal epithelium. In contrast to endometriosis the glands are not surrounded by endometrial stroma and there is no stromal hemorrhage.

Neoplasms of the Fallopian Tubes

The tumors of the fallopian tubes are relatively rare. These tumors may be benign or malignant. Malignant tumors may be primary in the fallopian tube or secondary owing to the metastasis or direct extension of malignant tumors from some other primary sites.

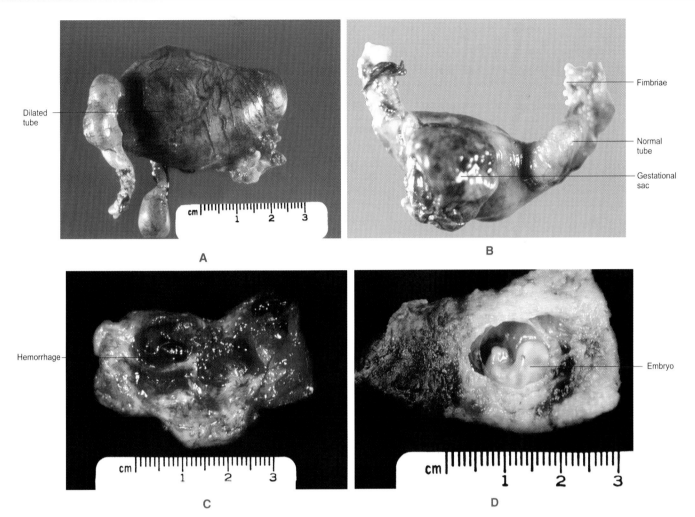

Figures 5.8A to D. Tubal pregnancy: A. The fallopian tube is dilated and contains a bluish-colored mass. B. The gestational sac has ruptured partially through the tubal wall. C. Cystic cavities, corresponding to dilated parts of the tubal lumen are filled with hemorrhagic tissue corresponding to placenta and remnants of the fetus. D. An embryo is identified in the gestational sac of tubal pregnancy.

1. *Adenomatoid tumor:* It is the most common benign tumor of the fallopian tubes. It is most often incidentally found during surgery performed for other reasons. It appears as a white or yellow nodule beneath the tubal serosa. The tumor originates from the mesothelium and is composed of tubules or gland-like structures permeating the muscle layer of the tubal wall (Fig. 5.10).

2. *Adenocarcinomas:* They rarely occur as primary tumors of the fallopian tubes. To qualify as a primary fallopian tube carcinoma, a tumor must be located within the tube or at the fimbriae end, and the uterus and ovary must not contain similar neoplasms. On gross examination, the tube is usually dilated and diffusely indurated or nodular. On cross section the tube is usually filled with papillary or solid tumor masses exhibiting areas of hemorrhage and necrosis. Invasion into the wall of the tube can be identified. Histologically, almost all malignant tumors of the fallopian tubes are adenocarcinomas. These tumors can be further classified as serous, mucinous, endometrioid or clear cell adenocarcinomas (Fig. 5.11). Some tumors have features of transitional cell carcinoma,

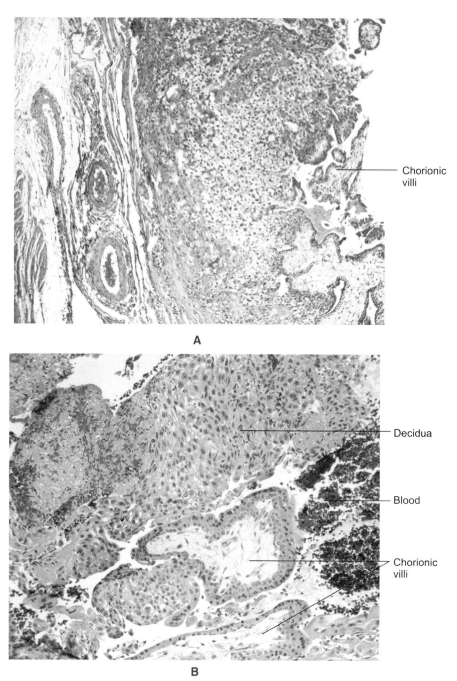

Figures 5.9A and B. Tubal pregnancy: A. Cross-section shows the presence of chorionic villi in the lumen of fallopian tube. B. Higher power view of the chorionic villi, decidua and clotted blood.

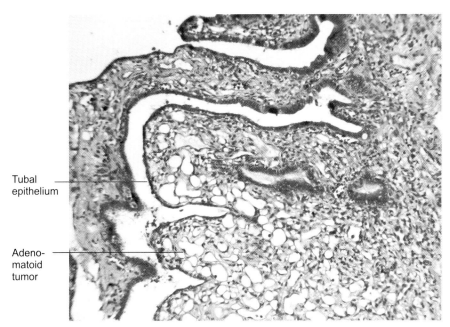

Tubal
epithelium

Adeno-
matoid
tumor

Figure 5.10. Adenomatoid tumor: The wall of fallopian tube contains a
mass composed of small tubules and gland-like structures.

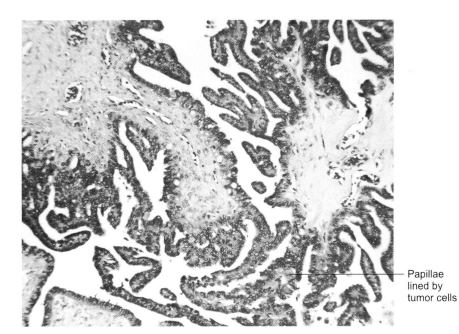

Papillae
lined by
tumor cells

Figure 5.11. Papillary serous carcinoma of the fallopian tube. Cuboidal
cells line connective tissue papillae that project into the lumen of the
fallopian tube.

and some are classified as undifferentiated carcinoma. These tumors are similar to ovarian or uterine carcinomas of the same histologic type.

3. *Metastatic carcinomas* involving the tube, usually originate from primary tumors in the ovary or endometrium. The spread of these tumors typically occurs by direct extension, but may also occur through the lymphatics, or by peritoneal implantation. Distant metastases from extrapelvic sites may also occur, but are less common.

Ovary

6

NORMAL ANATOMY AND HISTOLOGY

The ovaries are almond shaped paired organs located in the pelvic cavity laterally to the uterus. Each ovary is enclosed in a dense fibrous capsule, the tunica albuginea, and is held in place by an ovarian ligament.

Two zones are recognized on cross section of a normally functioning ovary (Fig. 6.1):

- *Cortex:* Composed of specific ovarian stroma, germ cells and follicles in various stages of growth and/or involution (Fig. 6.2).
- *Medulla:* Composed of nonspecific fibrous tissue and blood vessels

The most important aspects of normal histology of the ovary that are essential for the understanding of ovarian pathology are as follows:

- The surface of the ovary is covered by simple cuboidal epithelium known as *germinal epithelium*.

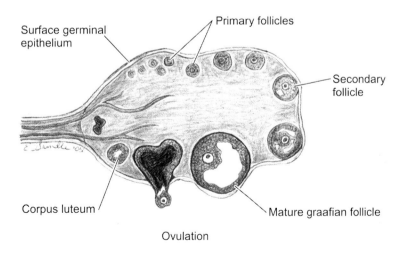

Figure 6.1. Ovary: Normal microscopic anatomy.

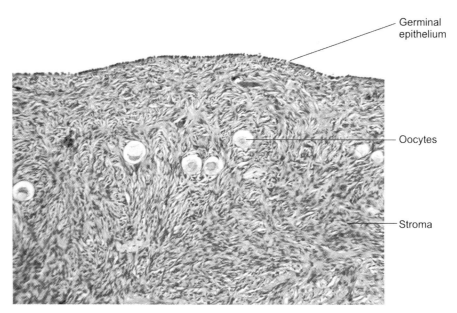

Figure 6.2. Cortex of the ovary: The stroma is compact and contains scattered primary oocytes. The surface of the ovary is covered by cuboidal germinal epithelium.

- At the time of ovulation, the surface epithelium ruptures and regenerates to cover the defect on the surface of the ovary. During this regeneration the epithelium may undergo neoplastic transformation and give rise to tumors. Suppression of ovulation by pregnancy or oral contraceptives is known to reduce the incidence of ovarian cancer.

• The germinal epithelium is derived from the *celomic epithelium* covering the fetal genital ridges.

- The celomic epithelium covering the genital ridges invaginates during fetal development. It gives rise to the mucosa of the müllerian ducts, i.e. the primordium of future fallopian tubes, endometrium, the cervix, and the upper part of the vagina. Ovarian tumors developing from the germinal epithelium may resemble epithelial lining of these organs. Accordingly, serous tumors resemble fallopian tube mucosa, mucous tumors resemble endocervical lining, and endometrioid tumors resemble endometrial mucosa. Brenner tumors are composed of transitional epithelium probably corresponding to the fetal epithelium of immature vagina.

• The cortex of the ovary contains numerous *germ cells*, which interact with sex cord cells to form *follicles* (Fig. 6.3).

- The germ cells are essential for the formation of follicles. In Turner's syndrome, a developmental disorder characterized by an early depletion of germ cells from the gonads, the ovaries transform during infancy and early childhood into fibrous gonadal streaks. Such gonadal streaks are devoid of follicles and hormone secreting sex cord cells.

- Ovaries depleted of oocytes at the time of menopause involute. Such ovaries do not contain follicles and do not secrete sex hormones.

• Follicles consist of oocytes and *sex cord cells: granulosa cells, theca interna* and *theca externa cells.*

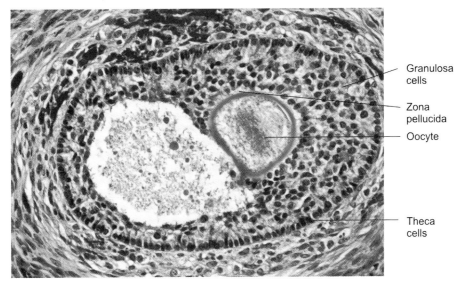

Figure 6.3. Maturing secondary follicle: The oocyte has a zona pellucida and is surrounded by granulosa cells. Around the corona of granulosa cells, one may see theca cells.

- The sex cord cells secrete steroid sex hormones, estrogens and progesterone. These cells also can give rise to female hormone producing tumors.
- After ovulation the follicle that has discharged the oocyte transforms into the *corpus luteum* (Fig. 6.4). Corpus luteum involutes and transforms into *corpus albicans*.
  - Follicles and corpora lutea may become cystic and persist secreting ovarian hormones in an abnormal pattern. Such cysts lead to enlargement of the ovaries and may be associated with menstrual or reproductive disturbances.
- The *hilum* of the ovary contains lipid rich *steroid secreting cells*, similar to the Leydig cells of the testis.
  - Steroid secreting cells of the hilum may give rise to hormonally active tumors causing virilization or hyperestrinism.

OVERVIEW OF PATHOLOGY

The most important diseases of the ovary include the following entities:
- Non-neoplastic cysts
- Endometriosis
- Neoplasms

Non-neoplastic Cysts

1. *Ovarian cysts:* They are derived from unruptured follicles or corpora lutea. They may be solitary or multiple (Box 6.1). Occasionally, attached to the ovary one may find solitary of multiple paraovarian cysts derived from remnants of incompletely involuted embryonic structures such as the mesonephros or the wolffian ducts.

Box 6.1. Ovarian and paraovarian cysts
- Solitary cysts
  - Follicular cysts
  - Corpus luteum cysts
- Polycystic ovary
- Paraovarian cysts

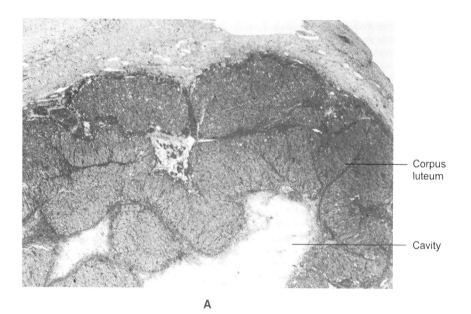

A

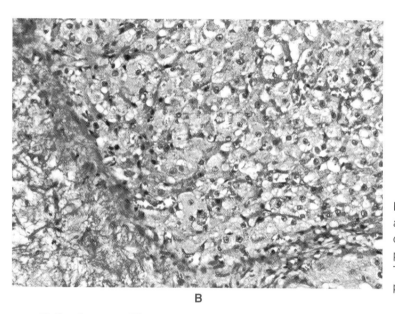

Figures 6.4A and B. Corpus luteum: A. It contains a central cavity surrounded by several layers of compacted granulosa lutein cells. B. Higher power view illustrating the granulosa lutein cells. These cells have abundant eosinophilic and partially vacuolated cytoplasm.

B

- *Follicular cysts:* They are the most common ovarian cysts. Most of them are small but occasionally they may enlarge even up to 10 cm in diameter (Fig. 6.5). Follicular cysts are lined by granulosa cells, that resemble cells forming normal follicles (Fig. 6.6). These cells also may show signs of luteinization. The cells acquire abundant eosinophilic cytoplasm thus mimicking normal follicular cells changing into luteinized cells.
- *Corpus luteum cysts:* They are derived from cystically dilated corpora lutea (Fig. 6.7). They often contain blood and have a thick yellow wall composed of luteal cells.
2. *Paraovarian cysts:* They are found on the surface of the ovary, in the mesoovary or mesosalpinx, and the broad ligament (Fig. 6.8). They are lined by cuboidal or flattened cells resembling normal mesothelium.
3. *Polycystic ovary:* It is typically found in women suffering from a complex disorder of the hypothalamic-pituitary-ovarian-adrenal hormonal known as polycystic ovarian disease (PCOD) (Box 6.2). The cortex of the ovary contains numerous follicular cysts (Fig. 6.9).

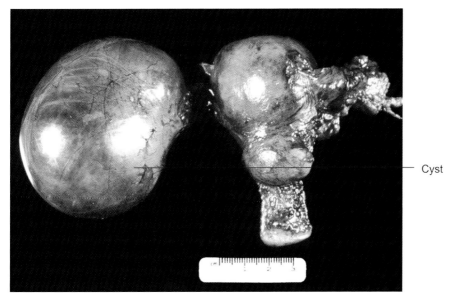

Figure 6.5. Follicular cyst: A large fluid filled cyst has almost completely replaced the ovary.

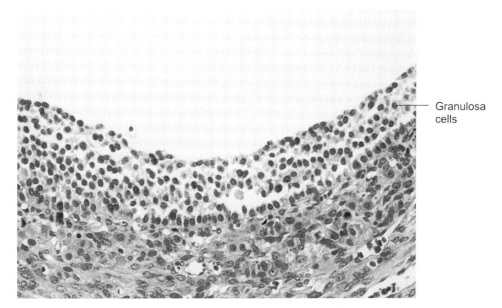

Figure 6.6. Follicular cyst: The lumen of the cyst is surrounded by slightly luteinized granulosa cells, and surrounded externally by theca cells.

Endometriosis

Endometriosis is a disease characterized by the presence of endometrial mucosa in extrauterine locations (Box 6.3). Most often it involves the ovaries, but it can be found anywhere in the abdominal cavity and in other extra abdominal sites (Box 6.4).

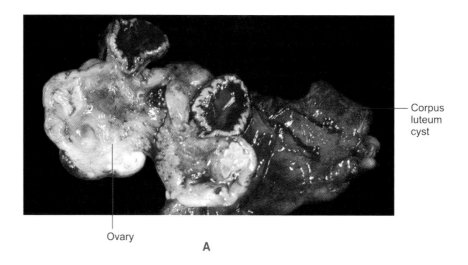

Corpus
luteum
cyst

Ovary

A

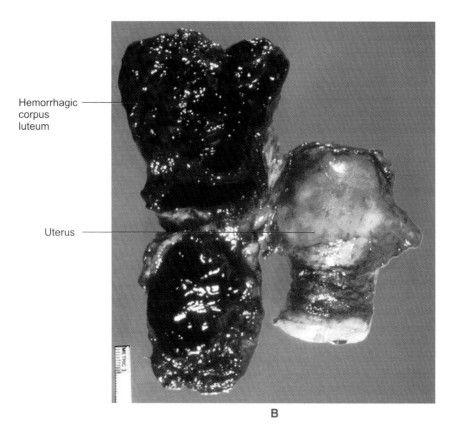

Hemorrhagic
corpus
luteum

Uterus

B

Figures 6.7A and B. Corpus luteum cysts: A. Bisected cystic corpus luteum filled with blood has a yellow wall composed of lipid-rich granulosa lutein cells. B. Hemorrhagic corpus luteum cyst contains clotted blood rimmed by a thin layer of brownish yellow tissue. The final diagnosis was made only upon histologic examination of the cyst wall.

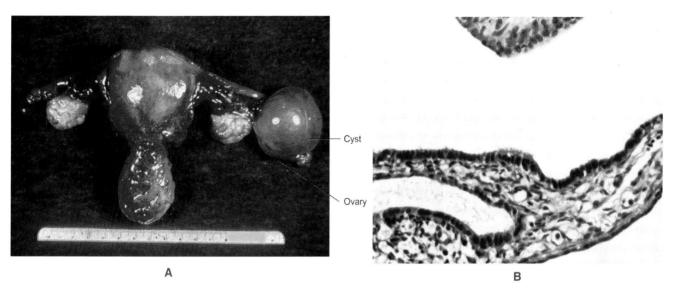

Cyst

Ovary

A

B

Figures 6.8A and B. Paraovarian cysts: A. The cyst is attached to the ovary. B. Microscopically, the cavities of the cyst are lined by flattened cuboidal epithelium.

Box 6.2. Clinical findings in polycystic ovary syndrome

SIGNS AND SYMPTOMS
- Menstrual disorders
  - Amenorrhea, oligomenorrhea
- Infertility
- Virilization
  - Hirsutism, acne and frontal alopecia
- Obesity

HORMONAL ABNORMALITIES*
- Androgens ↑
- Luteinizing hormone (LH) ↑
- Follicle stimulating hormone (FSH)↓

PATHOLOGY
- Bilateral polycystic ovaries
- Cysts lined by follicular cells

* Primary disorders of the pituitary and adrenal must be excluded

Box 6.3. Endometriosis

EPIDEMIOLOGY
- Prevalence 10 to 15% during reproductive age
- 80% of patients are 20 to 50 year-old
- 5% postmenopausal

CLINICAL FEATURES
- Pelvic pain
- Dysmenorrhea
- Infertility

PATHOLOGY
- Laparoscopic finding of red serosal spots
- Hemorrhagic nodules and masses
- Biopsy: Endometrial tissue

Box 6.4. The most common locations of endometriosis

- Ovaries
- Uterine ligaments
- Rectovaginal septum
- Pelvic peritoneum
- Laparotomy scars
- Peritoneum of other abdominal organs

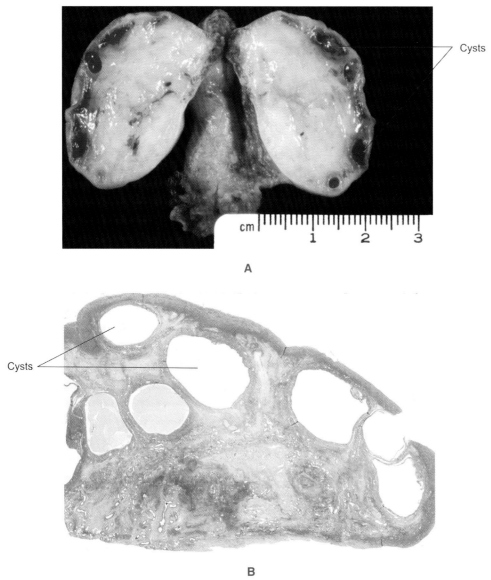

Figures 6.9A and B. Polycystic ovary: A. The cortex of the bisected ovary contains numerous small cysts. B. Microscopic cross-section through the ovary shows the cortical cysts.

It may present in form of multiple small hemorrhagic serosal spots. Large hemorrhagic masses or cysts filled with degraded blood ("chocolate cyst") may entirely destroy or obliterate the ovary (Fig. 6.10). Histologically, the foci of endometriosis are composed of endometrial glands and stroma and often contain central cavities filled with old blood (Fig. 6.11).

Neoplasms

For practical purposes ovarian neoplasms can be divided histogenetically into five major groups (Fig. 6.12):

- Surface epithelial-stromal tumors

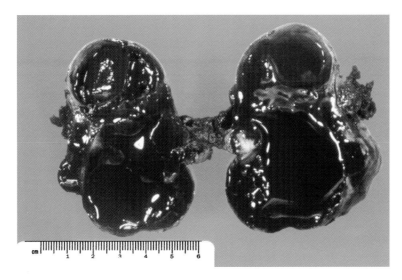

Figure 6.10. Endometriosis of the ovary: The bisected ovary contains a large blood filled cyst ("chocolate cyst").

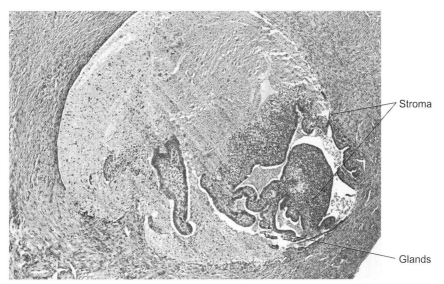

Figure 6.11. Endometriosis of the ovary: The central microscopic cavity lined by columnar epithelium contains old blood. The glands are rimmed by endometrial stroma.

- Germ cell tumors
- Sex-cord stromal tumors
- Tumors of uncertain origin
- Metastases from other organs.

Primary tumors represent 95% of all ovarian neoplasms. Metastases to the ovary account for the remaining 5% of neoplasms.

Surface Epithelial-stromal Tumors

These epithelial tumors originate from the germinal surface epithelium. However, since the tumors also contain typical cortical ovarian stroma it is more appropriate to include that term into their name.

Depending on the histologic appearance of the epithelial component these tumors are classified into several groups (Box 6.5). On gross examination they may be solid or cystic, unilateral or bilateral. Cystic tumors may be unilocular or multilocular. Clinicopathologically almost all of these groups comprise three subsets:

- Benign tumors
- Borderline tumors
- Malignant tumors.

Serous tumors: They are usually cystic and often papillary. These tumors are divided into three groups: benign serous cystadenomas, borderline serous tumors and malignant serous cystadenocarcinomas (Box 6.6).

Box 6.5. Surface-epithelial stromal tumors
• Serous tumor
• Mucinous tumor
• Endometrioid tumor
• Clear cell tumor
• Transitional cell tumor
• Squamous cell tumor
• Undifferentiated carcinoma
• Mixed epithelial tumor
• Malignant mixed müllerian tumor

Box 6.6. Serous tumors of the ovary			
Features	Cystadenoma	Borderline tumor	Cystadenocarcinoma
Frequency	60%	15%	25%
Bilaterality	15%	30%	65%
Age (years)	30-70 (peak 50)	30-50 (peak 45)	40-80 (peak 55)
5-year survival	100%	90-95%	Stage I-75%
			Stage II-55%
			Stage III-25%

1. *Serous cystadenomas:* They have a smooth external surface (Fig. 6.13A). A typical tumor consists of a solitary cyst or multiple thin-walled cysts filled with serous clear yellow fluid. Some cysts may contain solid nodules in their wall, associated with intracystic papillary protrusions. Such protrusions may be small wart-like or large resembling cauliflower. Histologically, the cysts of serous tumors are lined by columnar or cuboidal partially ciliated epithelium, reminiscent of the epithelial lining of the fallopian tubes (Fig. 6.13B). Benign serous tumors which have a more prominent fibrous stroma are called serous cystadenofibromas (Fig. 6.14).

2. *Serous borderline tumors (SBT):* They may on external examination resemble cystadenomas but often their internal surface may be covered with papillary outgrowth (Fig. 6.15). On cross sectioning, they are usually multicystic and often partially solid. The cysts typically contain numerous papillary protrusions or cauliflower-like nodules that have a velvety surface. The cysts contain a viscous fluid that may be mistaken for mucus. Histologically, the papillae projecting into the lumen of cysts show more complexity (Fig. 6.16A). The epithelium is multilayered, stratified and it may extend endophytically into the underlying stroma. Mild to moderate nuclear atypia is present, but the mitotic activity is not prominent. Tumors that show severe nuclear atypia are called *borderline serous tumors with intraepithelial carcinoma.*

   In contrast to overtly invasive cystadenocarcinomas, SBT do not show true destructive stromal invasion. Microinvasion of the stroma in form of small invasive cell nests or single cells is seen in 10% of SBT; these findings have no adverse prognostic significance (Fig. 6.17).

   In about one-third of all SBT there are microscopic or even macroscopically visible peritoneal implants measuring 1 to 2 cm in diameter. The histologic features of these implant vary. Some are exophytic and papillary, some resemble endosalpingiosis and some are invasive (Fig. 6.18). Histologically, such implants are classified as noninvasive (accounting for 90% of cases) or invasive, which are rare (Fig. 6.19).

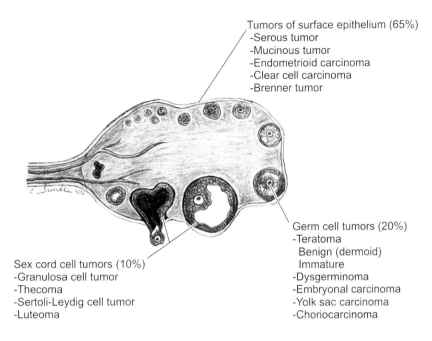

Tumors of surface epithelium (65%)
-Serous tumor
-Mucinous tumor
-Endometrioid carcinoma
-Clear cell carcinoma
-Brenner tumor

Germ cell tumors (20%)
-Teratoma
  Benign (dermoid)
  Immature
-Dysgerminoma
-Embryonal carcinoma
-Yolk sac carcinoma
-Choriocarcinoma

Sex cord cell tumors (10%)
-Granulosa cell tumor
-Thecoma
-Sertoli-Leydig cell tumor
-Luteoma

Figure 6.12. Histogenesis of primary ovarian tumors: Tumors may originate from the surface germinal epithelium, the germ cells, or the sex-cord stromal cells of the follicles.

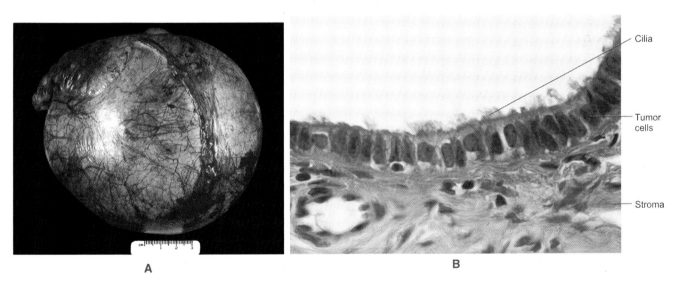

Cilia

Tumor cells

Stroma

A

B

Figures 6.13A and B. Serous cystadenoma: A. Tumor appears like a distended balloon because it is filled with fluid. The external surface is smooth and shiny. B. Microscopically, the cyst is lined by cuboidal or cylindrical cells that have uniform nuclei. Some cells are ciliated.

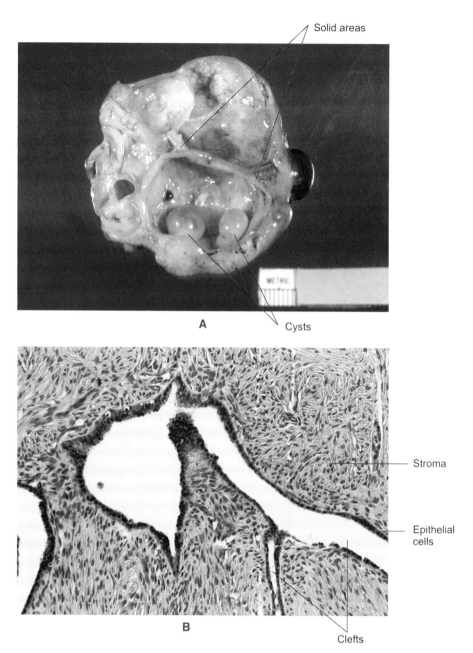

Figures 6.14A and B. Serous cystadenofibroma: A. This multicystic tumor contains broad solid areas. B. Microscopically, the tumor is composed of fibrous stroma lined along the clefted interior by a single layer of cuboidal cells.

3. *Serous cystadenocarcinomas:* These are partially cystic tumors with large solid components (Fig. 6.20). Papillary nodules may be seen inside the cystic cavities or on the external surface. Poorly differentiated tumors may present as solid masses. These tumors are bilateral in two thirds of patients and tend to metastasize through peritoneal seeding.

Microscopically, malignant serous tumors are usually high-grade adenocarcinomas. They show irregular branching of papillae lined by atypical stratified epithelium (Fig. 6.21). Small cellular papillae may fill the entire cavity of cystic

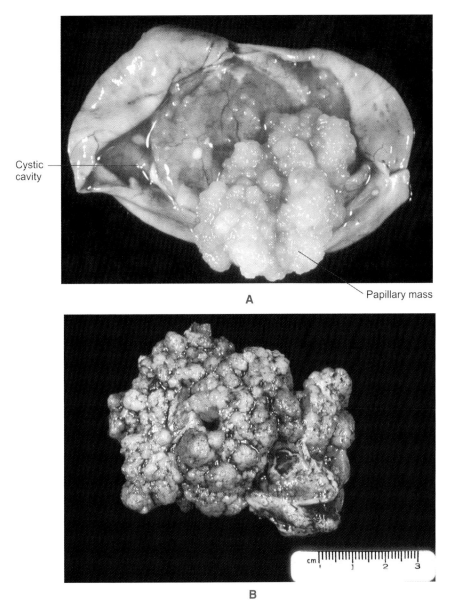

Figures 6.15A and B. Serous borderline tumors: A. Cystic tumor contains on its internal surface a cauliflower like papillary mass that has a velvety surface. B. This tumor has multiple papillary excrescences on its external surface.

tumors. Even in well-differentiated tumors there is unquestionable evidence of stromal invasion. Poorly-differentiated tumors consist of solid sheets of highly atypical malignant cells. Metastases are often found on the peritoneum and the peritoneal fluid contains tumor cells typically arranged into groups and forming papillary fronds (Fig. 6.22).

Mucinous tumors of the ovary: It can also be divided into three groups: benign mucinous cystadenomas (75%), borderline mucinous tumors (10%) and malignant mucinous cystadenocarcinomas (15%) (Box 6.7).

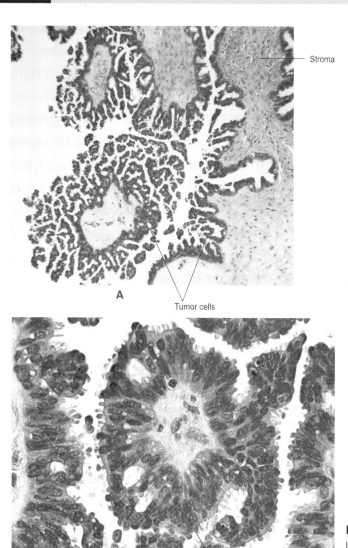

Stroma

Tumor cells

A

Tumor cells

B

Figures 6.16A and B. Serous borderline tumor: A. The lumen is lined by multilayered hyperchromatic epithelial tumor cells. B. Higher power view illustrating the atypia and multilayering of epithelial cells.

Box 6.7. Mucinous tumors of the ovary			
Feature	*Cystadenoma*	*Borderline tumor*	*Cystadenocarcinoma*
Frequency	75%	10%	15%
Bilaterality	5%	5-40%*	5%#
Age (years)	20-70 (peak 40)	20-70 (peak 50)	35-80 (peak 51-54)
5-year survival	100%	90%	Stage I-85%
			Stage II-55%
			Stage III- 20%

* Borderline tumors of the intestinal type are bilateral only in 5% of all cases; borderline endocervical type tumors are bilateral in 40% of all cases

Mucinous cystadenocarcinoma involving both ovaries are rare and most of such tumors represent metastases from the gastrointestinal tract

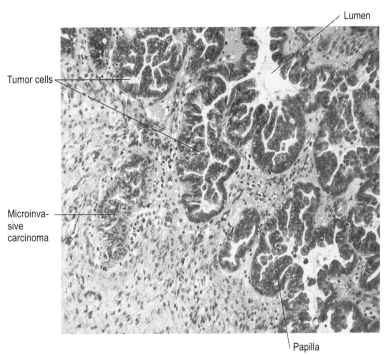

Lumen

Tumor cells

Microinvasive carcinoma

Papilla

Figure 6.17. Serous borderline tumor: Tumor cells line surface invaginations from the central cavity and also line papillae protruding into the lumen. Microinvasion is identified by the presence of tumor cell nests in the stroma. By definition such nests should not exceed 10 mm² in size.

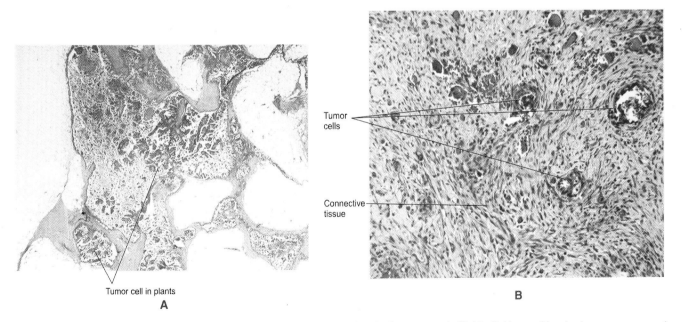

Tumor cell in plants

A

Tumor cells

Connective tissue

B

Figures 6.18A and B. Noninvasive peritoneal implants of serous borderline tumor. A. Epithelial type of implants are composed of glands enclosed in loose connective tissue under the surface of the peritoneal cavity. B. Desmoplastic type of implant consists of neoplastic glands surrounded by connective tissue.

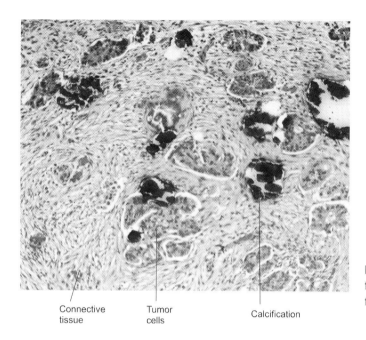

Connective tissue   Tumor cells   Calcification

Figure 6.19. Invasive peritoneal implant: Neoplastic cells form irregular groups located inside the clefts of fibrous tissue. In this case there are also calcifications.

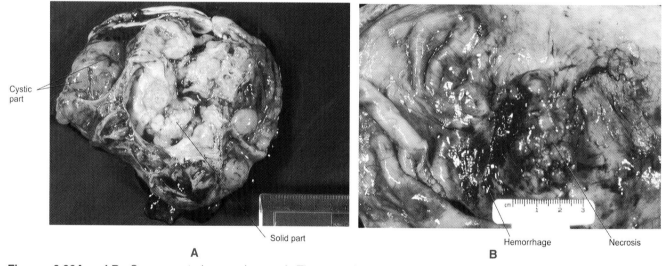

Cystic part

Solid part

A

Hemorrhage   Necrosis

B

Figures 6.20A and B. Serous cystadenocarcinoma: A. The tumor is mostly solid, but also contains some cystic parts. B. The inside of the cyst of this tumor contains hemorrhagic and partially necrotic nodules protruding into the central cavity.

1. *Mucinous cystadenomas:* These are usually large, cystic, unilocular or multilocular tumors filled with viscous mucus (Fig. 6.23). Mucinous cystadenofribomas may contain solid parts. Histologically, the tumor is lined by cylindrical or cuboidal mucin secreting cells with basally located nuclei showing no atypia.

2. *Mucinous tumors of borderline malignancy:* These are in 80% of all cases composed of a single large cavity with only a few smaller cysts in its wall (Fig. 6.24). Histologically, the cysts are lined by mucus secreting cells showing resemblance to endocervical or intestinal epithelium (Fig. 6.25). Tumor cells show nuclear atypia, crowding

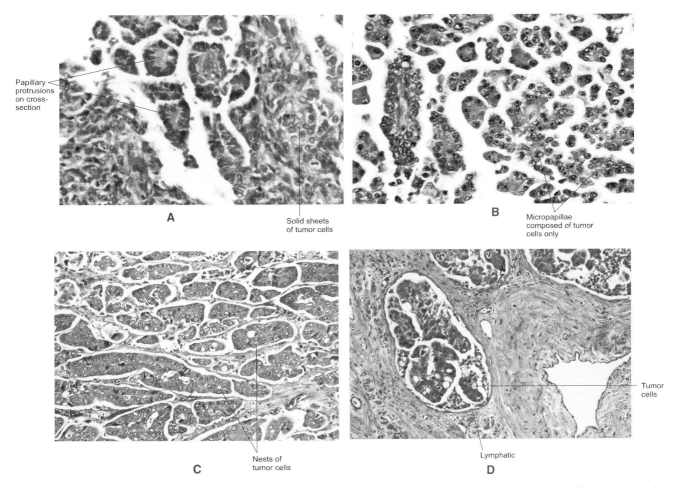

Figures 6.21A to D. Papillary serous cystadenocarcinoma: A. The inside of the cavity contains solid sheets of hyperchromatic neoplastic cells that also cover the papillary protrusions. B. Micropapillary adenocarcinoma is composed of small cells forming pseudopapillae that lack central fibrous cores. C. Invasive carcinoma in the wall of the tumor consists of cellular nests. D. Lymphatic spread of tumor cells.

and stratification along the papillary fronds, but no stromal invasion. In 10% of cases there are foci of microinvasion, which do not alter the diagnosis and do not influence the prognosis.

3. *Mucinous cystadenocarcinomas:* These are cystic tumors containing large mucoid solid parts (Fig. 6.26). Histologically they represent adenocarcinomas, which are in about 80% also contain remnants of mucinous cystadenoma or mucinous borderline tumor.

Mucinous cystadenocarcinomas may be indistinguishable histologically from metastatic adenocarcinoma from the gastrointestinal tract. Immunohistochemistry is used to distinguish primary ovarian mucinous tumors from metastases: ovarian tumors express cytokeratin 7 (CK7), whereas the metastases from the colon and rectum do not express CK7. In contrast, colorectal cancers express CK20, which is not expressed in ovarian mucinous adenocarcinomas. In some tumors it may be found but only focally and staining rather weakly.

Peritoneal metastases are associated with accumulation of mucus in the abdominal cavity. Such *pseudomyxoma peritonei* may occur in patients who have other mucinous tumors of the ovary as well. However, current evidence

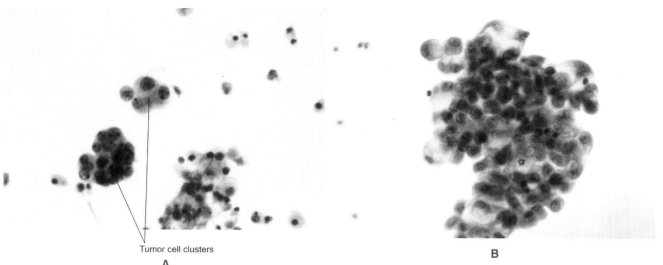

Tumor cell clusters

A

B

Figures 6.22A and B. Papillary serous cystadenocarcinoma: A. The cytologic smears prepared from the peritoneal wash contain clusters of tumor cells. B. The papillary nature of the tumor can be recognized even in cytologic smears.

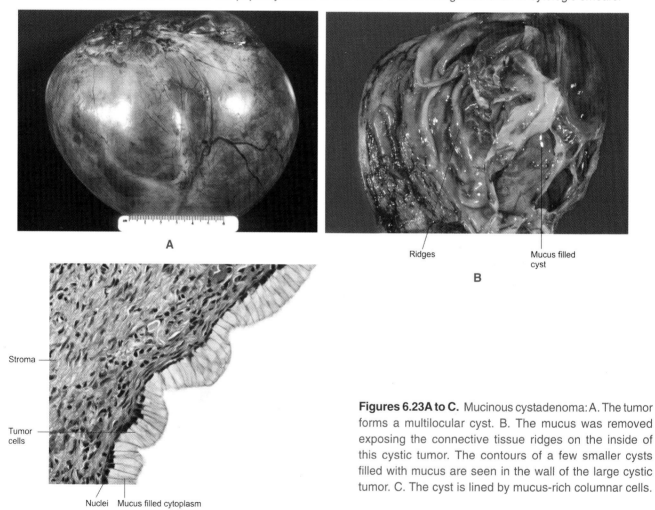

A

Ridges

Mucus filled cyst

B

Stroma

Tumor cells

Nuclei   Mucus filled cytoplasm

C

Figures 6.23A to C. Mucinous cystadenoma: A. The tumor forms a multilocular cyst. B. The mucus was removed exposing the connective tissue ridges on the inside of this cystic tumor. The contours of a few smaller cysts filled with mucus are seen in the wall of the large cystic tumor. C. The cyst is lined by mucus-rich columnar cells.

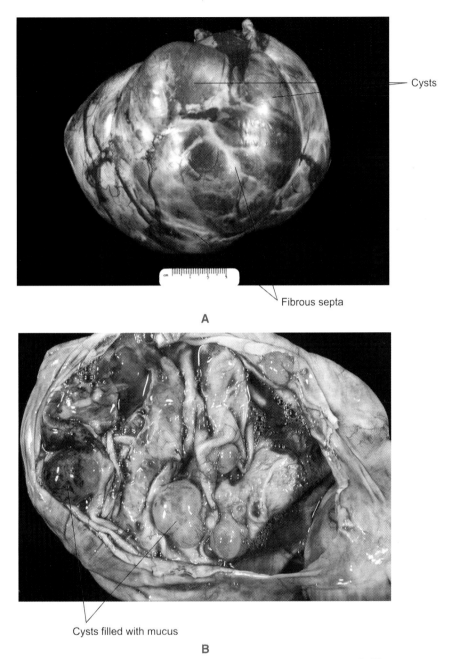

Cysts

Fibrous septa

A

Cysts filled with mucus

B

Figures 6.24A and B. Mucinous tumor of borderline malignancy: A. The tumor is multilocular and thus appears lobulated from outside. B. Upon opening of the cystic tumor one may see that it has a principal cavity and several smaller cysts attached to it.

indicates that most pseudomyxomas peritonei are of gastrointestinal origin and related to mucinous tumor of the appendix.

Endometrioid tumors of the ovary: They are also classified as benign, borderline and malignant. Benign endometrioid cystadenomas are rare, the criteria for borderline tumors are controversial, and accordingly endometrioid

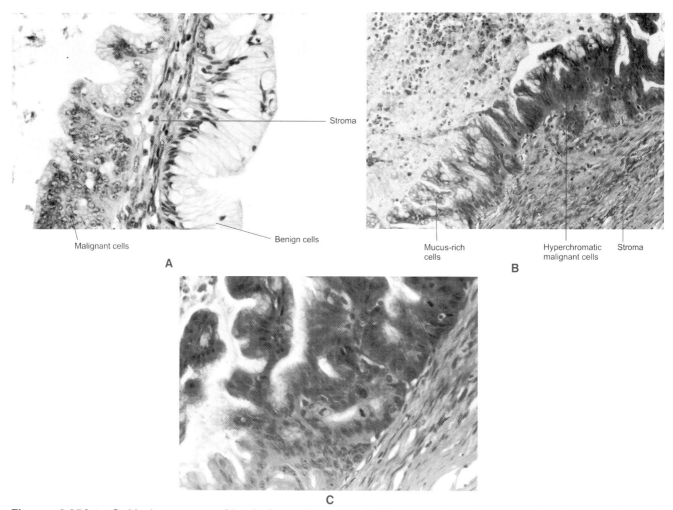

Figures 6.25A to C. Mucinous tumor of borderline malignancy: A. The hyperchromatic tumor cells show crowding and stratification. Compare the malignant cells with the benign mucinous cystadenoma cells on the right hand side. B. Hyperchromatic cells have almost completely lost mucus from their cytoplasm. C. Higher power view of hyperchromatic cells. Note that there is no invasion of the stroma.

adenocarcinomas are the only endometrioid tumors of any clinical significance. They represent 10 to 20% of all ovarian carcinomas.

Endometrioid adenocarcinomas are predominantly solid tumors (Fig. 6.27A). Approximately 40% of patients have also endometriosis and in 15 to 20% of cases there is a concomitant endometrial adenocarcinoma. Histologically they are composed of neoplastic gland like structures resembling endometrial adenocarcinoma (Fig. 6.27B).

Clear cell tumors of the ovary: They are almost invariably malignant; benign clear cell tumors are exceptionally rare and borderline malignant tumor account for less than that 1% of all borderline tumors. Clear cell carcinomas account for approximately 5% of all ovarian malignant tumors. They are typically found in older postmenopausal women.

Clear cell carcinoma may be entirely solid, but are more often partially cystic containing multiple solid nodules (Fig. 6.28). Histologically the tumors are composed of clear, eosinophilic or hobnailed cells arranged into tubulocystic or papillary structures, with frequent areas of consolidation (Fig. 6.29).

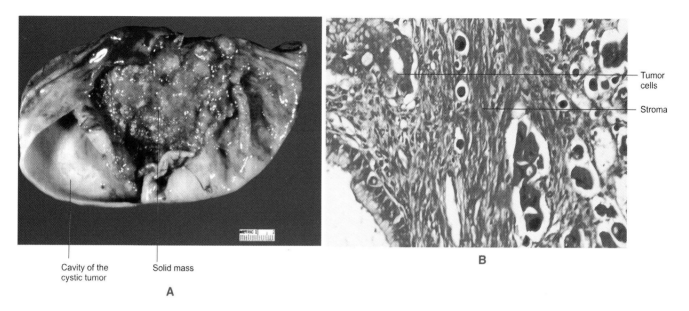

Cavity of the cystic tumor

Solid mass

A

Tumor cells

Stroma

B

Figures 6.26A and B. Mucinous cystadenocarcinoma: A. The tumor is cystic but contains a large solid mass that has a shiny appearance due to mucus pouring out from the cut surface. B. The tumor cells invade the stroma.

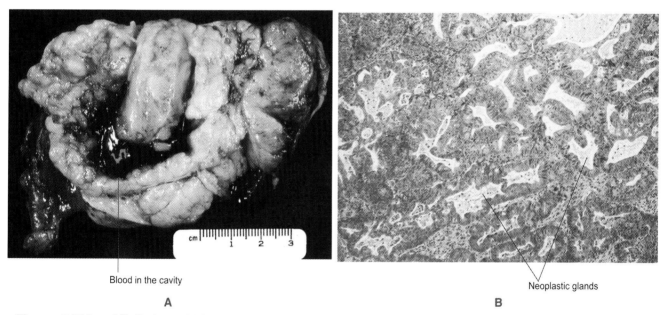

Blood in the cavity

A

Neoplastic glands

B

Figures 6.27A and B. Endometrioid carcinoma: A. The tumor is solid but contains a central cavity filled with clotted blood. B. Tumor is an adenocarcinoma resembling endometrial adenocarcinoma.

Benign transitional cell tumors are known as Brenner tumors. *Borderline malignant* and *malignant Brenner tumors* are rare. Likewise *transitional cell carcinomas* of the ovary are exceptionally rare.

Brenner tumors are common neoplasms but of limited clinical significance. Most tumors are small or even microscopic and found incidentally. Only 10% tumors are larger than 10 cm (Fig. 6.30). On cross-section such tumors appear solid, but in part they may be cystic. Histologically they are composed of nests of benign transitional epithelium surrounded by fibrous stroma.

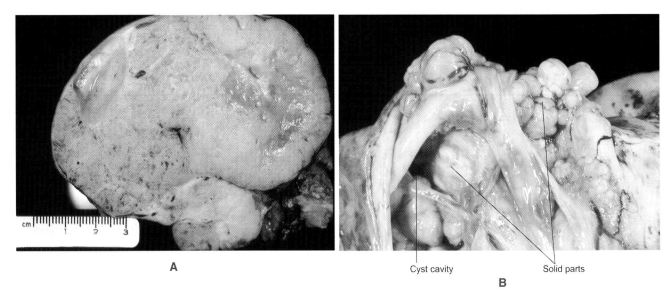

Figures 6.28A and B. Clear cell carcinoma: A. The tumor is solid grayish yellow. B. Another tumor is cystic but contains solid masses in its wall.

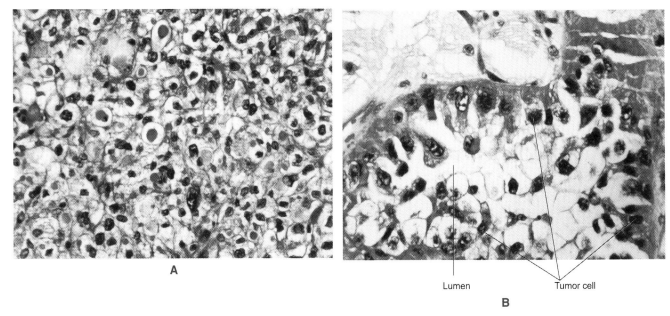

Figures 6.29A and B. Clear cell carcinoma: A. Tumor is composed of sheets of clear cells. B. Hobnailed and clear cells line tubulocystic spaces surrounded by fibrous septa.

Germ Cell Tumors

Germ cell tumors account for approximately 30% of all ovarian tumors. Approximately 95% of these tumors are classified as benign teratomas. The principal germ cell tumors are listed in Box 6.8 and the clinical features in Box 6.9.

Box 6.8. Germ cell tumors of the ovary

- Teratoma
- Dysgerminoma
- Yolk sac tumor
- Embryonal carcinoma
- Choriocarcinoma

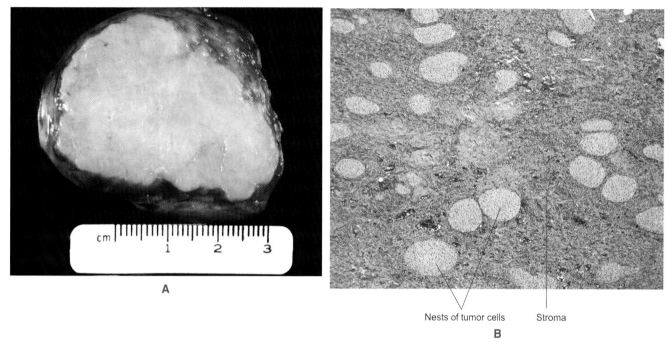

Nests of tumor cells   Stroma

B

Figures 6.30A and B. Brenner tumor: A. The cut surface of this solid tumor appears grayish white. B. Microscopically, the tumor is composed of nests of transitional epithelium surrounded by fibrous stroma.

Teratoma (dermoid cyst) It is a benign germ cell tumor composed of haphazardly arranged tissues derived from all three embryonal germ layers (ectoderm, mesoderm and endoderm). These tumors are typically cystic and composed predominantly of skin and its appendages (Fig. 6.31). The cyst usually contains sebum and hair. The lumen is typically lined by squamous epithelium, but the wall contains other tissues such as neural tissue, glands, cartilage, bone, or teeth. Clinical features are listed in Box 6.10.

1. *Secondary malignant transformation of teratomas:* It occurs in tumors that are left *in situ* untreated for long time. Such tumors may give rise to squamous cells carcinoma, or less commonly to neuroendocrine tumors (e.g. carcinoids), or even sarcomas.

2. *Immature teratomas:* They are tumor of children and adolescents. In addition to mature somatic tissues such tumors contain immature fetal neural tissue. These tumors are usually solid and may metastasize by peritoneal seeding (Fig. 6.32). Accordingly they are malignant.

Box 6.9. Germ cell tumors

EPIDEMIOLOGY
- 30% of all ovarian tumors
- 75% in women younger than 30 years

CLINICAL FEATURES
- Benign (95% are teratomas!)
- Usually unilateral
- Malignant variants respond well to chemotherapy
- Malignant tumors have serologic markers (hCG and AFP)

Box 6.10. Teratomas

EPIDEMIOLOGY
- The most common germ cell tumor
- Most patients < 30 years

CLINICAL FEATURES
- Palpable ovarian mass
- X-ray shows calcification of teeth
- No hormonal symptoms
- No serologic tumor markers
- Benign in most cases
- Immature teratomas—malignant
- Malignant transformation—rare complication in older women

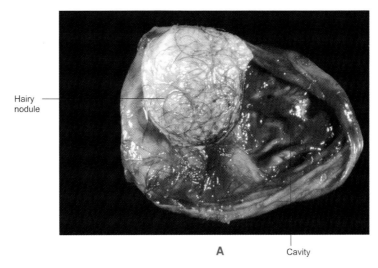

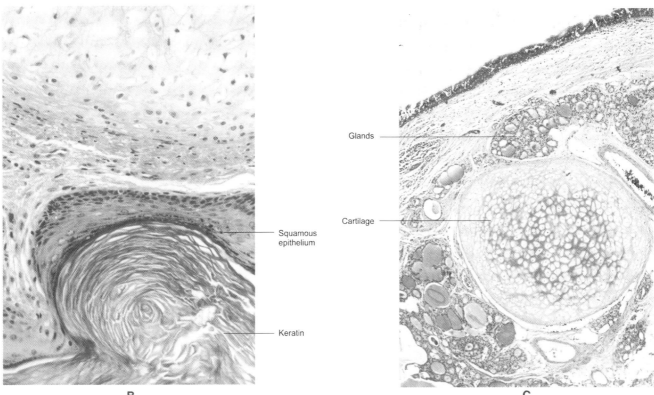

Figures 6.31A to C. Teratoma: A. The tumor is cystic but contains on its internal surface a nodule partially covered with hair. B. Microscopically the cavity is lined by keratinizing squamous epithelium. C. The wall of the tumor contains cartilage and glands.

3. *Monodermal teratomas:* They are tumors that show selective overgrowth of some components. Among these tumors the best known is *struma ovarii,* a tumor composed predominantly of thyroid tissue (Fig. 6.33).

Dysgerminoma It is equivalent to the seminoma of the testis (Fig. 6.34). It is the most common nonteratomatous germ cell tumor and it accounts for 50% of all malignant germ cell tumors.

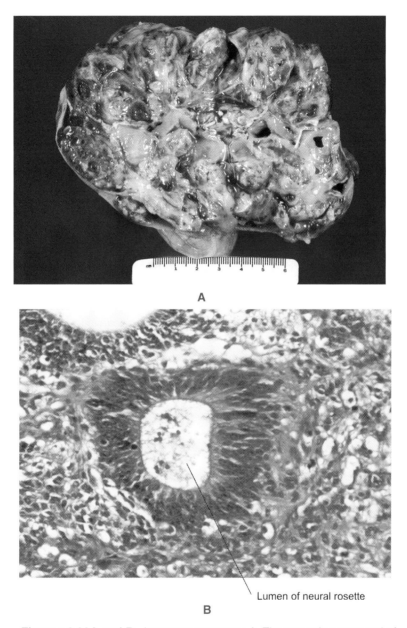

Lumen of neural rosette

Figures 6.32A and B. Immature teratoma: A. The tumor is composed of friable solid tissue. B. The tumor contains immature fetal neural cells arranged into neural rosettes.

Embryonal carcinoma is composed of malignant embryonal cells. *Yolk sac carcinoma* is composed of structures that resemble fetal yolk sac (Fig. 6.35). It secretes alpha fetoprotein (AFP), which appears in the blood and is a useful tumor marker. Choriocarcinoma is composed of cytotrophoblastic and syncytiotrophoblastic cells, resembling choriocarcinoma of the uterus or testis. Trophoblastic cells secrete chorionic gonadotropin, which is a useful diagnostic tumor marker. Approximately 5 to 10% of tumors contain more than one component and are classified as *mixed germ cell tumors*.

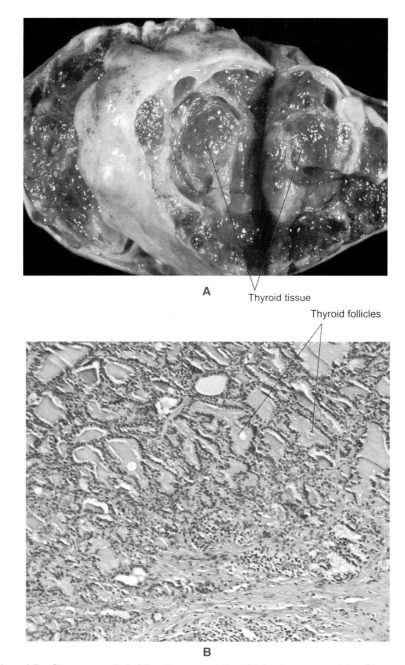

Figures 6.33A and B. Struma ovarii: A. Like the normal thyroid the tumor consists of brown tissue. B. Microscopically the tumor consists of thyroid follicles filled with eosinophilic colloid.

Sex-cord Stromal Tumors

Sex-cord stromal tumors (SC-ST) account for less than 10% of all ovarian tumors. This group contains a number of hormonally active tumors, but some of them may be nonfunctional (Box 6.11). Fibroma-thecoma group accounts for over 85% of all sex-cord stromal cell tumors, granulosa for 10%, whereas all others are rare.

Box 6.11. Sex-cord stromal tumors

- Fibroma
- Thecoma
- Granulosa cell tumor
- Sertoli-Leydig cell tumor
- Sclerosing stromal tumor
- Steroid cell tumor

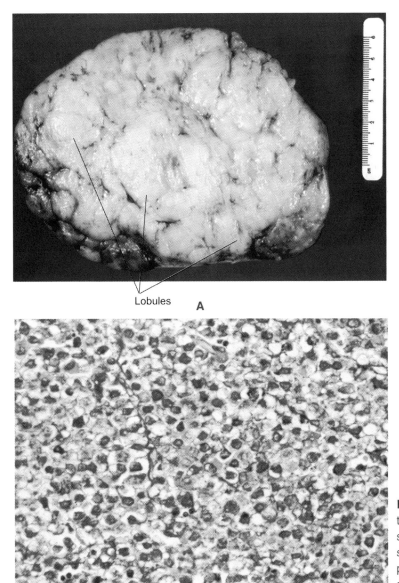

Lobules A

B

Figures 6.34A and B. Dysgerminoma: A. The tumor is lobulated, solid and on cross section appears grayish-yellow. B. Microscopically the tumor is composed of polygonal clear cells arranged into solid sheets.

Fibroma: It is a tumor composed of fibroblasts enclosed in collagenous extracellular matrix. The tumor is solid, firm and grayish yellow on cross section (Fig. 6.36). Histologically the tumor is composed of spindle-shaped fibroblastic cells and abundant collagen. Fibromas do not secrete hormones, but may be associated with ascites or pleural effusion (Meigs' syndrome). *Fibrosarcoma,* the malignant equivalent of fibroma is rare, but even so, it represents the most common ovarian sarcoma (Box 6.12).

Box 6.12. Fibroma of the ovary

EPIDEMIOLOGY
- The most common SC-ST of ovary
- Any age group (peak 55 years)

CLINICAL FEATURES
- Incidental palpatory finding
- Often calcified
- Bilateral 10%
- Hormonally inactive
- Ascites in 20% cases
- Meigs syndrome (1%)

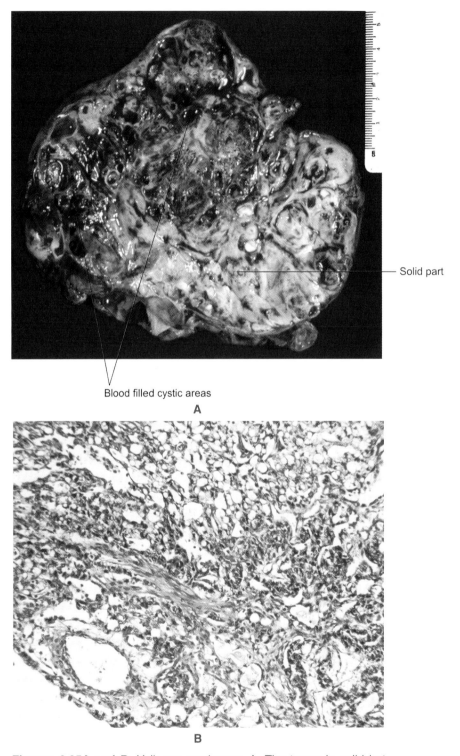

Solid part

Blood filled cystic areas

A

B

Figures 6.35A and B. Yolk sac carcinoma: A. The tumor is solid but contains also cystic areas filled with blood. B. Microscopically the tumor cells are arranged into several patterns. One may see cords, tubules, microcysts, solid nests, and micropapillary structures.

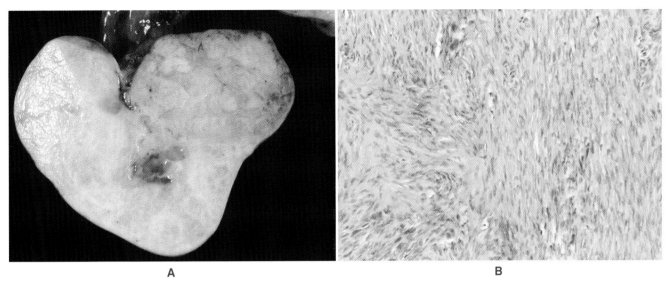

A B

Figures 6.36A and B. Fibroma: A. The solid tumor appears grayish white on cut surface. B. Tumor is composed of fibroblasts enclosed in collagenous matrix.

Thecoma: It is a tumor composed of lipid rich theca cells and luteinized cortical stromal cells as well as fibroblasts (Fig. 6.37). Special stains (e.g. oil red O) are useful for demonstrating cytoplasmic fat droplets in tumor cells. Luteinized cells are especially prominent in so-called *luteinized thecoma.* Typically tumors are solid, firm and on cross section appear yellow. Microscopically and macroscopically thecomas show an overlap with ovarian fibromas. Thecomas are invariably benign (Box 6.13).

Granulosa cell tumor It occurs in two distinct forms: adult granulosa cell tumor (AGCT) (95% of all tumors) that is typically found in postmenopausal women, and juvenile granulosa cell tumor (5% of all tumors) that is found in children and young adults. AGCT is the most common estrogen-secreting tumor of the ovary. On gross examination the tumor is solid, vaguely lobulated with focal cystic areas often containing hemorrhagic zones (Fig. 6.38). On cross sectioning it is grayish yellow.

Histologically it is composed of spindle shaped cells with typical "coffee bean-like" grooved nuclei. Tumor cells form solid masses, nests, cords or microfollicular structures resembling Call-Exner bodies.

Clinically all AGCT have a malignant potential (Box 6.14). Overall the prognosis is however good since most tumors are diagnosed in stage I, which has a 5-year survival of over 85%.

Box 6.13. Thecoma

EPIDEMIOLOGY
- Peak incidence in postmenopausal women
- Luteinized thecoma-30% in young women

CLINICAL FEATURES
- Unilateral ovarian mass (>95%)
- Estrogen secretion
- Vaginal bleeding (60%)
- Endometrial adenocarcinoma (20%)

Box 6.14. Granulosa cell tumor

EPIDEMIOLOGY
- Most common estrogenic tumor
- Adult type: Peak in 50-55 years age group
- Juvenile type: Children and adolescents

CLINICAL FEATURES
- Dysmenorrhea or amenorrhea
- Vaginal bleeding (postmenopausal)
- Unilateral ovarian mass
- Rupture→hematoperitoneum (10%)
- Good prognosis for stage I tumors
- Potential metastases even many years after surgery

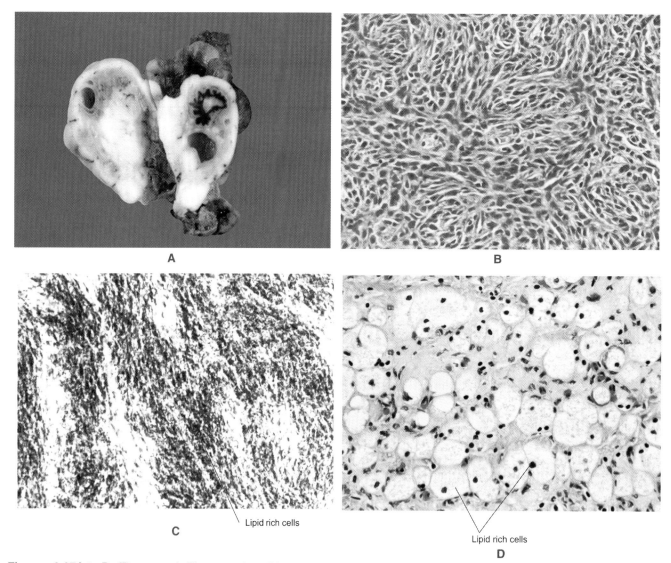

A

B

C

Lipid rich cells

Lipid rich cells

D

Figures 6.37A to D. Thecoma: A. The tumor is solid and its cut surface is yellow. B. Microscopically the tumor is composed of whorls of spindle shaped cells. C. Oil red O stain show that the tumor cells contain lipid droplets (red). D. Lipid rich cells are prominent in so called luteinized thecoma.

Sertoli-Leydig cell tumor It is a rare ovarian tumor composed of cells resembling Sertoli and stromal-interstitial cells of the testis. It is the most common virilizing tumor of the ovary. The tumor is solid, lobulated and grayish yellow on cross sectioning (Fig. 6.39). Large tumors composed of undifferentiated cells maybe necrotic and hemorrhagic.

Histologically the tumor is biphasic and consists of Sertoli cells arranged into tubules or cords or nests and groups of spindle stroma cells, or cells resembling Leydig cells. These cells have well-developed eosinophilic cytoplasm and round nuclei. Several histologic subtypes are recognized. Some tumors contain heterologous elements such as cartilage, hepatic tissue or mucin secreting glands. Tumors are graded as well-differentiated, intermediately and poorly-differentiated (Box 6.15).

Box 6.15. Sertoli-Leydig cell tumor

EPIDEMIOLOGY
- Rare tumor
- Young women (peak age 25 years)

CLINICAL FEATURES
- Menstrual disturbances
- Virilization (up to 50% patients)
- Unilateral ovarian mass
- Prognosis excellent except a few poorly differentiated tumors

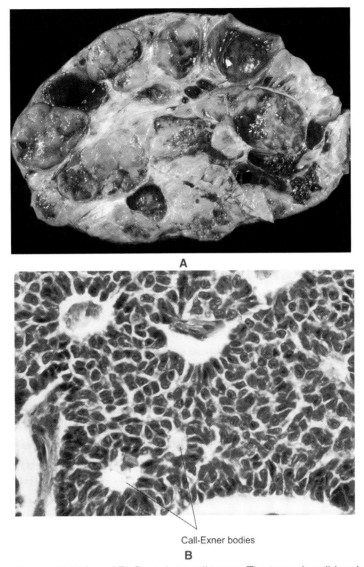

Call-Exner bodies

B

Figures 6.38A and B. Granulosa cell tumor: The tumor is solid and appears yellowish-tan on cut surface. B. Granulosa cells have coffee bean-shaped nuclei and form microfollicular structures corresponding to Call-Exner bodies in graafian follicles.

Steroid cell tumors: These are rare tumors composed of lipidized cells corresponding to hilar cells, Leydig cells, luteinized stromal cells or adrenal cortical cells. Several subtypes are recognized. The most common is the *steroid tumor, Not Otherwise Specified (NOS)*. On gross examination the tumor is solid and yellow on cross section (Fig. 6.40). Microscopically it is composed of solid sheets of polygonal cells with round nuclei and abundant eosinophilic or vacuolated and clear cytoplasm. These tumors are mostly benign but approximately 30% are malignant. Clinical features are listed in Box 6.16.

Box 6.16. Steroid cell tumor, NOS

EPIDEMIOLOGY
- Rare tumor
- Middle aged women (peak 45 years)

CLINICAL FEATURES
- The most common steroid cell tumor
- Dysmenorrhea/amenorrhea/infertility
- Androgenic (50%)
- Estrogenic (10%)
- Malignant 30%

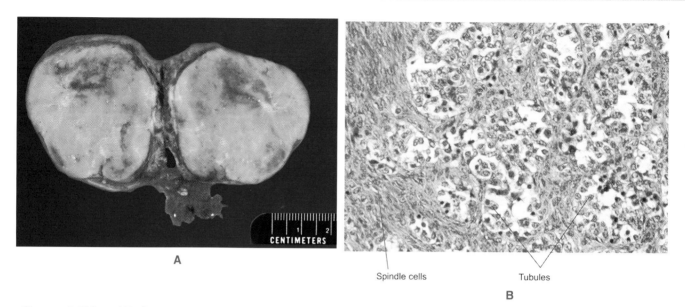

Figures 6.39A and B. Sertoli-Leydig cell tumor: A. Tumor is solid and appears yellow tan on cut surface. B. Microscopically, the tumor is biphasic and composed of cuboidal cells forming tubules and spindle cells around them.

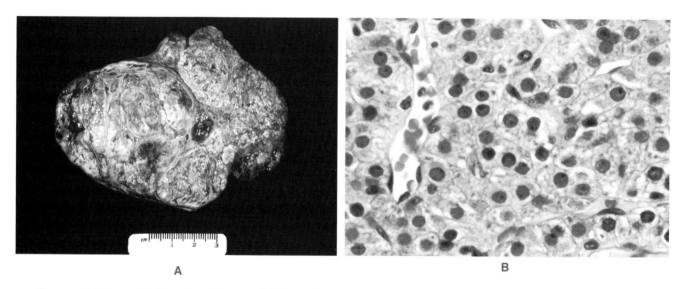

Figures 6.40A and B. Steroid cell tumors: A. This malignant tumor appears multilobulated and yellow on cut section. B. Microscopically, the tumor is composed of polygonal cells with round nuclei and well-developed cytoplasm.

Metastases to the Ovaries

Even though metastases account only for 5% of all ovarian tumors, the ovary is nevertheless the most common metastatic site in the female genital system. The most common primary tumors that metastasize to the ovaries are listed in Box 6.17.

Gastric carcinoma tends to involve both ovaries and present as a *Krukenberg tumor*. Ovaries are enlarged and have a smooth external surface

Box 6.17. Primary sites of tumors metastatic to the ovaries

- Gastrointestinal tract
- Endometrium
- Breast
- Lymph nodes/bone marrow (Lymphoma and leukemia)

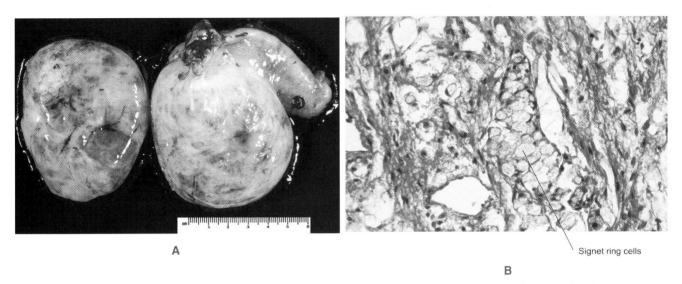

A

B
Signet ring cells

Figures 6.41A and B. Krukenberg tumor: A. Both ovaries are enlarged but have a smooth external surface. B. Microscopically, the ovary is infiltrated with signet ring carcinoma cells.

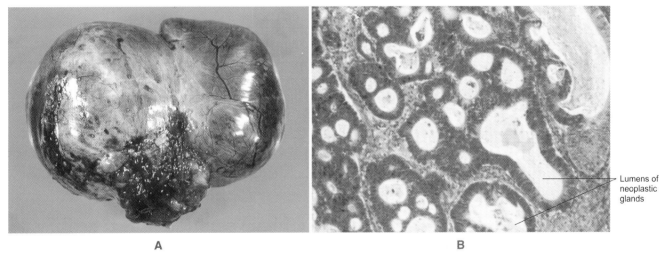

Lumens of neoplastic glands

A   B

Figures 6.42A and B. Colorectal carcinoma metastasis to the ovary. A. The tumor is a cystic mass entirely replacing the ovary and thus resembles a primary ovarian mucinous cystadenocarcinoma. B. Microscopically, the tumor is an adenocarcinoma composed of neoplastic glands lined by columnar cells.

(Fig. 6.41). Histologically the stroma of the ovary is permeated with signet-ring mucin rich tumor cells that form cords or nests or grow as single cells.

Colorectal carcinoma also tends to metastasize to both ovaries. Such metastases form cystic or partially solid masses resembling mucinous cystadenocarcinomas (Fig. 6.42). Microscopically the tumors are mucin-secreting adenocarcinomas, which often show typical central necrosis. Immunohistochemistry is used to distinguish such metastases from primary ovarian mucinous adenocarcinomas.

7

Placenta

NORMAL ANATOMY AND HISTOLOGY

Normal placenta is an organ that exists only during pregnancy. It has several main parts which include the umbilical cord, fetal membranes (amnion and chorion), placental disc composed of villous parenchyma, and maternal decidua (Fig.7.1). The normal term placenta weighs 450 to 600 gm and measures 15 to 20 cm in diameter.

1. *Umbilical cord:* It contains three vessels (two arteries and a single vein) that are embedded within a highly mucoid connective tissue called Wharton's jelly. The umbilical cord may insert in the placenta centrally or eccentrically. The site of cord insertion is usually *central* or *eccentric*, and occasionally *marginal* or *velamentous* (insertion into the fetal membranes) (Fig. 7.2). The significance of marginal insertion is uncertain, but velamentous insertion is associated with fetal anomalies, fetal loss or increased incidence of prematurity.

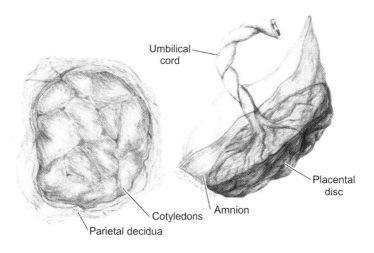

Figure 7.1. Normal placenta

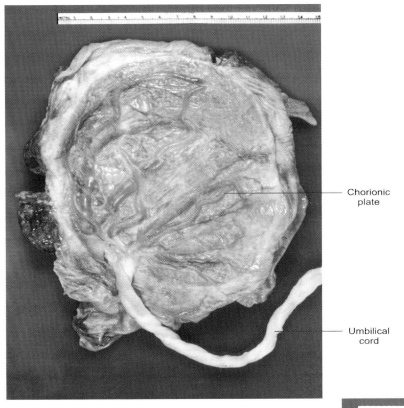

Chorionic
plate

Umbilical
cord

A

Cotyledons

B

Figures 7.2A and B. Marginal insertion of the umbilical cord (Battledore). A. Chorionic plate, which is smooth and glistening is facing the fetus. B. The basal plate is coarse and subdivided into cotyledons. The cord is inserted into one of the margins of the placental disc.

2. *Fetal membranes:* These consist of the amnion, which represents the most inner covering of the amniotic cavity, and the chorion, which is composed of a membranous connective tissue carrying the fetal vasculature. Normally, the fetal membranes insert along the margins of the placental disc. If the fetal membranes insert onto the placental disc more centrally and away from the margins a *circumvallate placenta* is formed (Fig. 7.3).

3. *Placental disc:* It is on the fetal side (*chorionic plate*) covered with amnion, whereas on the uterine side (basal plate) is coarsely lobulated and subdivided into smaller subunits called cotyledons. Occasionally it may be bilobed or separated into several lobes (*multilobate placenta*) (Fig. 7.4). In twin or triplet pregnancies the placental disc may be common for both fetuses or subdivided into two or three parts. These parts may fuse together into a large irregularly shaped placental disc (Fig. 7.5).

4. *Chorionic villi of the placental disc:* They constitute the functional units of the placenta. Each villus has a central mesenchymal core containing fibroblasts, blood vessels and scattered macrophages. Externally villi are covered by trophoblastic cells (Fig. 7.6).

   Trophoblastic cells include cytotrophoblastic, syncytiotrophoblastic cells and intermediate trophoblastic cells. The *cytotrophoblastic cells* form the inner layer on the surface of the villi, where the outer layer is formed of multinucleated *syncytiotrophoblastic cells* (Fig. 7.7). As the placenta matures, the cytotrophoblast becomes less conspicuous, and the syncytiotrophoblastic cells are clumped into "syncytial knots". These cells produce human chorionic gonadotropin (hCG). The cells of the *intermediate trophoblast* are found mostly in the extravillous region and form the deepest structural component of placenta at the implantation site. These cells produce human placental lactogen (hPL)

5. *Decidua:* It represents the gestational endometrial stroma. It is present on the placental disc as well as on the chorionic side of the membranes.

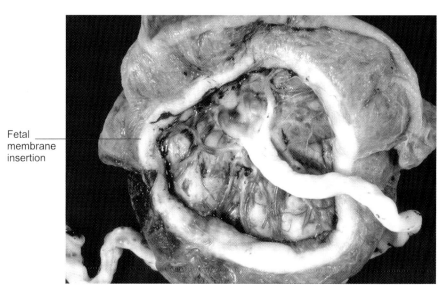

Fetal
membrane
insertion

Figure 7.3. Circumvallate placenta: The fetal membranes insert
centripetally from the peripheral margin.

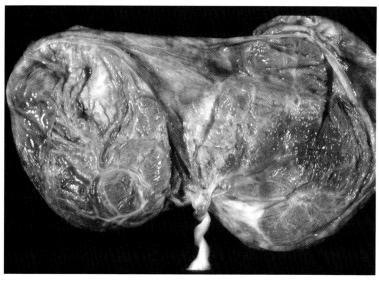

Figure 7.4. Bilobed placenta: The placenta consists of two lobes which are separated one from another by membranous chorion. The umbilical cord is connected to both lobes.

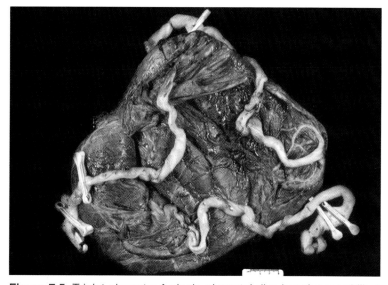

Figure 7.5. Triplet placenta: A single placental disc has three umbilical cords. All the fetuses were in one amniotic cavity and thus this placenta was termed monochorionic monoamniotic.

OVERVIEW OF PATHOLOGY

The most important diseases of the placenta are:

- Infections
- Disturbances of implantation and separation of the placenta
- Gestational trophoblastic disease.

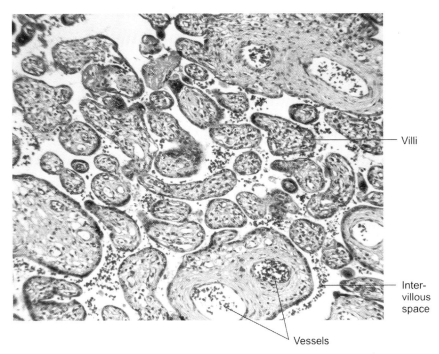

Villi

Inter-villous space

Vessels

Figure 7.6. Chorionic villi from term placenta. Each villus has a connective tissue core with blood vessels and is covered on its surface with trophoblastic cells.

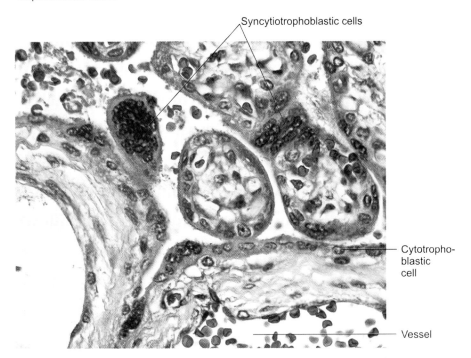

Syncytiotrophoblastic cells

Cytotropho-blastic cell

Vessel

Figure 7.7. Trophoblastic cells from term placenta. The villi are covered with mononuclear cytotrophoblastic cells and multinucleated syncytiotrophoblastic cells.

Infections

Placental inflammation presents usually as *acute chorioamnionitis* (Fig. 7.8), *acute funisitis* (Fig.7.9) or *villitis* (Fig. 7.10) Chorioamnionitis is most often caused by bacterial ascending infection (Box 7.1). Villitis may be caused by ascending infections or hematogenous infections with bacteria, viruses, protozoa or fungi (Box 7.2).

Disturbances of Implantation and Separation

Normal implantation typically occurs inside the uterine cavity. In some instances it may occur in the lower segment over the cervical canal. Such implantation (*placenta previa*) is accompanied by hemorrhage during pregnancy and an increased incidence of preterm deliveries.

1. *Extrauterine pregnancies:* These occur most often in the fallopian tubes. Tubal pregnancies account for over 95% of all extrauterine pregnancies. Ovarian, pelvic or abdominal pregnancies are less common.

2. *Abnormal intrauterine implantation:* It may due to incomplete formation of the decidual layer. In such cases the chorionic villi adhere to the myometrium or invade it preventing normal separation of the placenta and the uterus at the time of the delivery. It may occur in several forms as follows:

- *Placenta accreta*: It is characterized by firm attachment of the placenta or parts of the placenta to the myometrium. There is however no invasion of the myometrium.
- *Placenta increta*: It is associated with invasion of chorionic villi into the myometrium.
- *Placenta percreta*: It is characterized by deep invasion of the myometrium by chorionic villi, which penetrated through the entire wall of the uterus.

3. *Retroplacental hematomas and placental abruption:* They represent the most important disturbances of separation of the placenta from the pregnant uterus. These conditions are not associated with any diagnostic pathologic changes.

Gestational Trophoblastic Disease

Gestational trophoblastic disease is a term for a heterogeneous group of disorders including abnormal development of the placenta, proliferation and in some cases even neoplastic transformation of trophoblastic cells. The most important diseases included in this group are as follows:

- Complete hydatidiform mole
- Partial hydatidiform mole
- Choriocarcinoma
- Placental site trophoblastic tumor.

1. *Complete hydatidiform mole:* It results from androgenesis, i.e. abnormal development of the fertilized ovum that has lost the maternal chromosomes and contains only the paternal chromosomes (Fig. 7.11). Since the paternal set of chromosomes reduplicate, complete moles have a 46,XX karyotype in most instances. Placental

Box 7.1. Chorioamnionitis and funisitis—most common causes

- *Mycoplasma hominis*
- *Ureaplasma urealyticum*
- *Bacteroides* sp.
- *Streptococcus agalactiae* (group B)

Box 7.2. Villitis—most common causes

- Bacteria
  - *Mycoplasma hominis*
  - *Chlamydia trachomatis*
  - *Treponema pallidum*
  - *Listeria monocytogenes*
- Viruses
  - Cytomegalovirus
  - Herpesvirus
  - Parvovirus
- Protozoa
  - *Toxoplasma gondii*

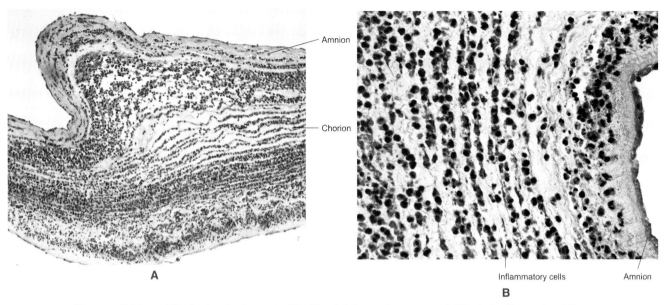

Amnion

Chorion

Inflammatory cells   Amnion

A

B

Figures 7.8A and B. Acute chorioamnionitis: The fetal membranes are infiltrated with neutrophils.

Blood vessel   Umbilical stroma

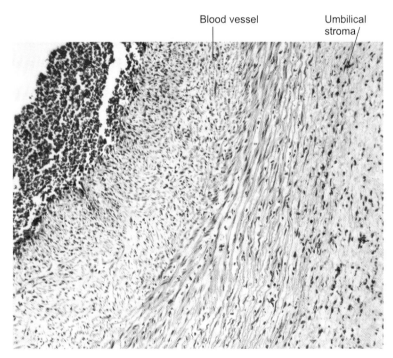

Figure 7.9. Acute funisitis: The umbilical cord is infiltrated with neutrophils, which also permeate the wall of the umbilical vessel.

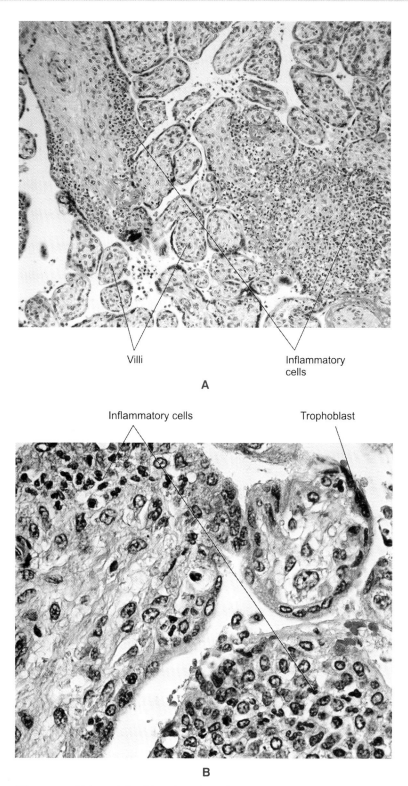

Villi   Inflammatory
cells

A

Inflammatory cells   Trophoblast

B

Figures 7.10A and B. Chronic villitis: Chorionic villi are infiltrated with chronic inflammatory cells destroying focally the trophoblastic surface layer.

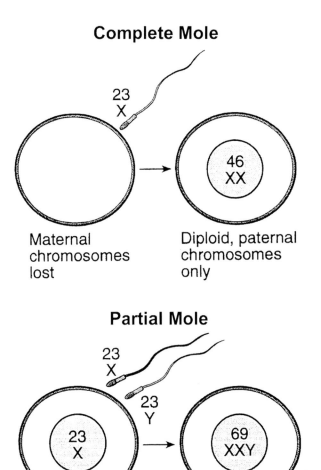

Figure 7.11. Pathogenesis of hydatidiform mole: Complete mole develops due to androgenesis. In this process the sperm contributes 23 paternal chromosomes. During or shortly after fertilization the maternal chromosomes die off. The paternal chromosomes reduplicate and the mole accordingly has a normal diploid number of chromosomes (46,XX). Incomplete mole develops after super fecundation with two spermatozoa. Since each sperm brings into the ovum 23 chromosomes, and the maternal set of chromosomes persists intact, the mole will contain 69 (i.e. 3 × 23) chromosomes. The karyotype of incomplete moles is 47,XXY or 47,XXX. The fetus develops but dies after 10 weeks of pregnancy.

chorionic villi transform into grape-like vesicles filled with fluid (Fig. 7.12). Histologically, these villi are edematous and expanded (Fig. 7.13). The villi are avascular and lined by hyperplastic trophoblast (Fig. 7.14). The fetus does not develop, and the molar pregnancy ends in a spontaneous abortion usually in the first trimester of the pregnancy.

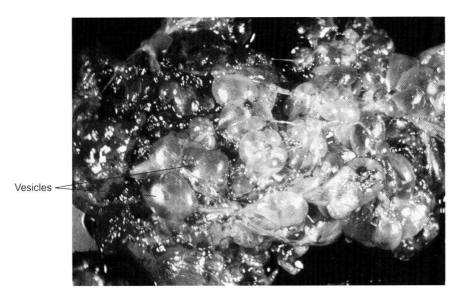

Figure 7.12. Complete hydatidiform mole: The chorionic villi have undergone transformation into grape-like vesicles.

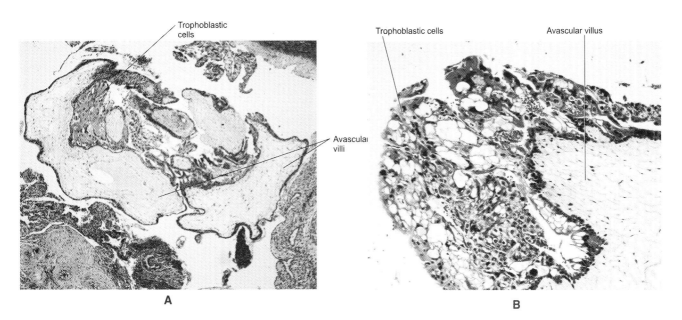

Figures 7.13A and B. Complete hydatidiform mole: A. The molar villi are avascular and edematous .On their surface the villi are lined by hyperplastic trophoblastic cells. B. Hyperplastic cytotrophoblastic cells and numerous syncytiotrophoblastic cells form solid nests.

2. *Partial hydatidiform mole:* It results from superfecundation with two spermatozoa, each of which contributes to the fertilized ovum one set of 23 chromosomes. Accordingly, the karyotype of molar cells is 69,XXY, or 69,XXX. The fetus, which usually dies after 10 weeks of pregnancy, can be found on gross examination. However, quite often it is not visible macroscopically (Fig. 7.14). Microscopically, two populations of chorionic villi are seen. Some villi are normal and some are avascular and swollen. Villi are usually invaginated and less edematous than in complete mole (Fig. 7.15). The trophoblastic proliferation is also less prominent and often only focal.

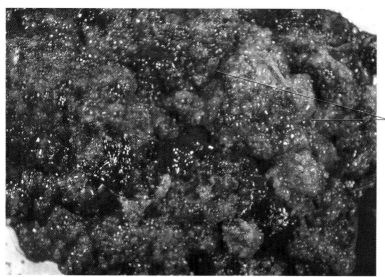

Figure 7.14. Partial hydatidiform mole: The placental chorionic villi have in part transformed into vesicles. Parts of the fetus were seen microscopically, but could not be identified with certainty on gross examination.

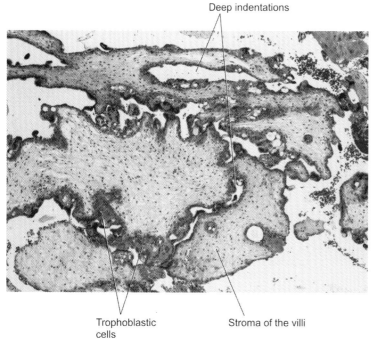

Figure 7.15. Partial hydatidiform mole: The chorionic villi are of irregular shapes and show deep indentations on their surface. The edema is less prominent than in complete mole and the trophoblastic proliferation is only focal.

3. *Choriocarcinoma:* It is a malignant tumor originating from placental tissue. The tumor is highly invasive and destructive (Fig. 7.16) and tends to metastasize hematogenously to the lungs, or the brain and other organs. Microscopically it is composed of neoplastic cytotrophoblastic and syncytiotrophoblastic cells (Fig.7.17).

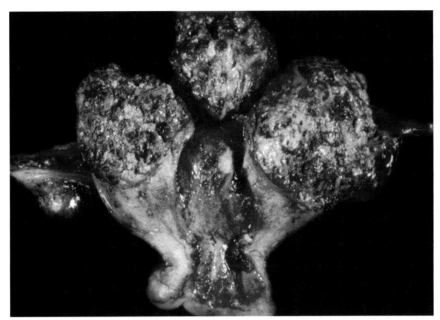

Figure 7.16. Choriocarcinoma: An invasive tumor, partially necrotic and hemorrhagic tumor is found in the upper part of the uterine cavity.

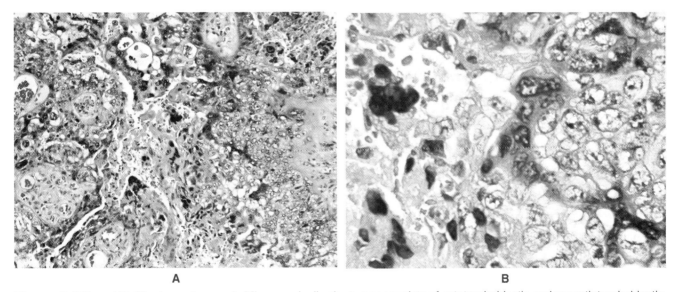

A   B

Figures 7.17A and B. Choriocarcinoma: A. Microscopically, the tumor consists of cytotrophoblastic and syncytiotrophoblastic cells. B. Higher power view of mononuclear cytotrophoblastic cells and multinucleated syncytiotrophoblastic cells.

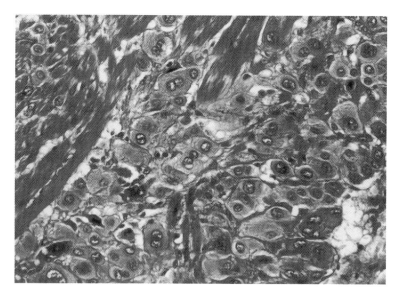

Figure 7.18. Placental site trophoblastic tumor: The tumor is composed of intermediate trophoblastic cells invading the myometrium.

4. *Placental site trophoblastic tumor:* It is a benign locally invasive tumor composed of intermediate trophoblast. Microscopically it resembles an exaggerated implantation site composed of columns of intermediate trophoblast invading into the myometrium (Fig. 7.18). Most tumors of this type respond to conservative therapy, but occasionally they may be more aggressive and atypical and require chemotherapy.

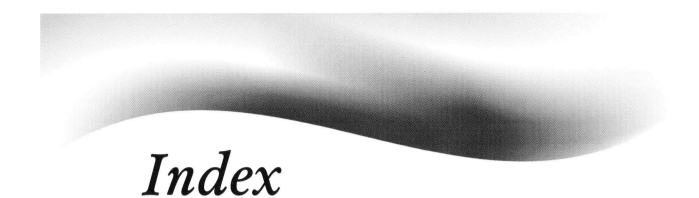

Index

WP
160
3/08.